Praise for *The Healing Touch for Cats*

"The long list of benefits—enhancing health, accelerating healing, increasing love and trust—must be experienced to be believed. Massage is something every pet owner should offer their pets, and this book has everything you need to get started."
—Susan Wynn, DVM, author of *Emerging Therapies: Using Herbs and Nutraceuticals*

"The world-renowned veterinarian Michael W. Fox shares his years of wisdom and insights regarding the world of hands-on healing and holistic medicine for our Kindred Spirits. Read it and help heal your animal friends!" —Allen Schoen, MS, DVM, author of *Kindred Spirits: How the Remarkable Bond between Humans and Animals Can Change the Way We Live*

"Dr. Michael Fox generously shares his twenty years of experience....Our pets' pain dissipates as the world of energetic vibrational healing comes alive on the pages of this easy-to-use book."
—Donna Kelleher, author of *The Last Chance Dog and Other True Stories of Holistic Animal Healing*

"A unique feature of these books is Dr. Fox's holistic viewpoint, which addresses not only the physical but also the mental, emotional, and spiritual aspects of pets' well-being and our relationships with them." —Jean Hofve, DVM

"Michael Fox provides feline owners with in-depth information to insure the physical and psychological well-being of their cats. Easy to follow guidelines for healing touch, massage therapy, natural healing and general health make *The Healing Touch for Cats* a book I would highly recommend." —Ann N. Martin, author of *Food Pets Die For: The Shocking Facts About Pet Food*

OTHER TITLES BY MICHAEL W. FOX

Canine Pediatrics

Integrative
Development of Brain
and Behavior in the
Dog

Canine Behavior

Concepts in Ethology,
Animal and Human
Behavior

Understanding Your Pet

Returning to Eden:
Animal Rights and
Human Responsibility

How to Be Your Pet's
Best Friend

Love Is a Happy Cat

The Healing Touch for
Dogs

Farm Animals:
Husbandry, Behavior,
and Veterinary
Practice (A Critic's
Viewpoint)

One Earth, One Mind

Behavior of Wolves,
Dogs, and Related
Canids

The Whistling Hunters

Between Animal and
Man: The Key to the
Kingdom

Laboratory Animal
Husbandry

The New Animal
Doctor's Answer Book

The New Eden

St. Francis of Assisi,
Animals, and Nature

Inhumane Society: The
American Way of
Exploiting Animals

Superdog: Raising the
Perfect Canine
Companion

Supercat: Raising the
Perfect Feline
Companion

You Can Save the
Animals: 50 Things
You Can Do Right
Now

Understanding Your
Dog

Understanding Your Cat

The Soul of the Wolf:
Observations and
Meditations

Superpigs and
Wondercorn: The
Brave New World of
Biotechnology and
Where It All Might
Lead

Agricide:The Hidden
Crisis That Affects Us
All

The Boundless Circle

Eating with Conscience:
The Bioethics of Food

Concepts in Ethology:
Animal Behavior and
Bioethics

Beyond Evolution: The
Genetically Altered
Future of Plants,
Animals, the Earth
...and Humanity

Bringing Life to Ethics:
Global Bioethics for a
Humane Society

Children's Books

Vixie, the Story of a
Little Fox

The Wolf

Sundance Coyote

Ramu and Chennai

What Is Your Dog
Saying? (with Wende
Devlin Gates)

What Is Your Cat
Saying? (with Wende
Devlin Gates)

Wild Dogs Three

Whitepaws: A Coyote-
dog

Lessons from Nature:
Fox's Fables

The Touchlings

The Way of the
Dolphin

Animals Have Rights,
Too

THE HEALING TOUCH FOR CATS
The Proven Massage Program

*(Formerly titled: Dr. Michael Fox's
Massage Program for Cats and Dogs)*

DR. MICHAEL W. FOX
D.Sc., Ph.D., B. Vet. Med., M. R. C. V. S.

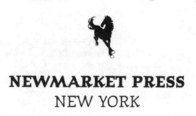

NEWMARKET PRESS
NEW YORK

To all my four-legged friends,
patients, teachers, and healers.

This book was originally published in hardcover by Newmarket Press as *Dr. Michael Fox's Massage Program for Cats and Dogs*.

Also available *The Healing Touch for Dogs*.

10 9 8 7 6 5 4 3 2 1

ISBN 1-55704-575-5

Library of Congress Cataloging-in-Publication Data

Fox, Michael W., 1937-
  The healing touch for cats : the proven massage program / Michael W. Fox.
      p. cm.
Rev. ed. of: Dr. Michael Fox's Massage program for cats and dogs, 1981. Includes bibliographical references and index.
  ISBN 1-55704-575-5 (pbk.)
  1. Cats—Diseases—Alternative treatment. 2. Massage for animals. I. Fox, Michael W., 1937- Dr. Michael Fox's Massage program for cats and dogs. II. Title.
  SF985.F68 2003
  636.8'089372—dc22
                                    2003025510

QUANTITY PURCHASES

Companies, professional groups, clubs, and other organizations may qualify for special terms when ordering quantities of this title. For information, write Special Sales Department, Newmarket Press, 18 East 48th Street, New York, NY 10017; call (212) 832-3575; fax (212) 832-3629; or e-mail mailbox@newmarketpress.com.

www.newmarketpress.com

Photo and illustration credits: All photos by Bill Crandall and illustrations by Miyoko Yamashita, except photos on pages 6 and 80 by Kevin McGuinness, illustrations on page 101 and photos on pages 108 and 128 by Machiko, illustrations on pages 103 and 105 courtesy of Tallgrass Publishers, and photo on page 120 by Karen Hatt.

Printed in the United States

Design by Kevin McGuinness

FOREWORD

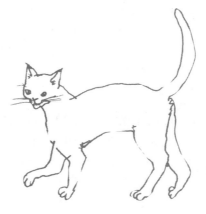

Since the first edition of this book was published more than twenty years ago, I have seen its ripple effect on the human-animal bond and on the quality of care and consideration people give to their animal companions.

We generally make physical contact with our animal companions quite unconsciously, and our enjoyment mirrors theirs while they are being "petted," which they will often solicit themselves. But when we touch them knowingly and make contact with specific parts of their bodies and at the same time consciously direct our energy, the Healing Touch is awakened. While "petting" helps affirm the human-animal bond, the Healing Touch is far more profound. Many readers have written to me confirming this observation. Shy animals have become more trusting; hyperactive and "neurotic" ones more calm. Aged and chronically ill animals have been given a new lease on life, or at least been made to feel more secure and comforted; and others have benefitted from their owners recognizing early signs of disease, since massage therapy is both diagnostic and therapeutic.

But as I emphasize in the book, massage is not a panacea. It is an adjunctive form of therapy and is one aspect of holistic healing that often entails a change in diet and other treatments rather than relying exclusively upon antibiotics, steroids, and other potentially harmful drugs. Many veterinarians who now practice holistic healing have found this book useful in their treatment programs; it's something they can give to their clients with very beneficial results. Several human massage therapists and massage therapy schools have also used *The Healing Touch* to help their clients and students apply the basic techniques to their animal companions.

Those who have discovered their own healing powers through touch, some after following the instructions in this book, should share their discovery with others. Certainly there is a lingering cultural taboo against touching others—even animals—that has to be overcome. Also the prejudice against the ancient healing arts will be encountered in those who are still enchanted by modern hi-tech "mechanistic" medicine and who are suspicious of any reference to the spiritual realm and to the higher power. Fear is the final barrier to be overcome before we can experience the essential unity of all sentient life. As a culture we have become as disconnected from the natural world as we have from our own natural senses and latent powers. Rediscovering the Healing Touch and applying it in the form of massage therapy to our friends—human and non-human alike—will do much to reconnect us all, for in wholeness is health. The Healing Touch, like the power of prayer in the laying on of hands, is a low-cost (often free) and very safe complementary and alternative medicine that we can all discover, practice, and enjoy giving and receiving.

Michael W. Fox
Washington, D.C.

CONTENTS

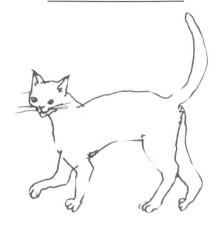

List of Diagrams

INTRODUCTION

I first became convinced of the "miracles" of massage for pets when I was studying wolf behavior in 1970 and had to treat one of my research wolves for distemper virus encephalitis—a serious inflammation of the brain. The animal was very sick and not responding to the usual methods of treatment. My prior experience with dogs who had this disease had always been negative, and at college we were taught to put such animals to sleep. But something in me refused to give up. It was then, acting out of desperation, a strong hunch, and the rewarding experiences I'd had with massage on people, that I decided to try massage on the ailing wolf.

I was, naturally, quite cautious at first, massaging almost tentatively and very gently and ever on the lookout for responses. The wolf seemed to enjoy being stroked and spoken to in a quiet reassuring voice. To begin with, I lightly massaged the muscles around her neck and head that were tense and frequently going into spasms. She responded positively by relaxing and going to sleep, but she was growing weaker by the hour, and the spasms were spreading and tremors shooting down her limbs. So I massaged her limbs and then applied deep-pressure massage up and down her spine. This seemed to energize and relax her, and for five days and nights I continued to massage her at intervals of every two or three hours for about fifteen minutes. Imagine my joy and satisfaction to see that the massage was producing healthful results!

Her recovery was complicated by the fact that she had a partial paralysis of her hind legs. She would give me different signals with her head when she wanted water or needed to be stood up to evacuate. I had to empty her bladder manually for several days. But with regular massage each day—especially of her hind legs and back—she regained control, and her muscle tone returned. Some residual hind-leg weakness persisted, but she compensated for this well.

The story has a happy ending. The wolf recovered with no treatment other than injections of glucose saline and phenobarbital to control seizures. She lived on for another eight active years, delivering a healthy litter of pups a few months after recovering from her near-fatal disease.

Subsequently, I used massage successfully on many occasions. My patients included cats and dogs with a variety of problems ranging from a generalized lack of vitality, convalescence, and old age to specific problems, such as arthritis, sprains, and recovery from surgery or broken limbs. Based on the perspective I gained from these cases, from my own experience, and from sound medical theory, I have come to believe in massage as an essential part of holistic pet health care—the new frontier in pet treatment.

I am sure that you have by now heard and read the word "holistic" often, and that you are aware of the holistic health movement, which is burgeoning everywhere. What do we mean when we speak of holistic health care?

Holistic is derived from the Greek word *holos*, which sounds very much like our own English word for it: "whole." Very simply, the holistic health approach aims to treat the body as a whole—the sum of its physical and psychological pieces—rather than to treat each part separately. The holistic doctor does not concentrate on treating the ailing leg, liver, lung, etc., but views the ailments in relation to the total human being or animal. This means that the holistic physician takes into consideration the effects of psychological stress, nutrition, exercise, and lifestyle, as well as viruses, bacterial infection, and organic malfunctioning.

I believe that pet massage is an essential part of total pet health care and maintenance. It is also more than that. It is not only a healthy measure and a healing tool, but it helps bring pet and owner closer. It is an amazing vehicle of communication and communion.

Until the advent of the holistic health movement, massage had been largely neglected in human health care and totally neglected in pet health care. That is because both animal and human medicine have become increasingly drug-oriented and depersonalized. But I think that it will soon be considered wrong for animal doctors to continue to indiscriminately prescribe drugs, such as antibiotics and steroids, as part of a treatment regimen that does not address the underlying causes of disease and only treats symptoms. Often drugs have harmful side effects, especially when treatment is prolonged and the condition chronic. Doctors have been criticized severely for practicing this kind of symptom-oriented, drug-dependent medicine.

I'm not opposed to the appropriate use of drugs and medical technologies. These are as much an integral part of holistic therapy as are massage and good nutrition. Neither the former nor the latter are panaceas, except for quacks and charlatans.

Today, massage and good nutrition should be part of holistic preventive medicine and health maintenance. Many pets tend to be obese and unexercised, just like their owners who do not practice right living themselves—over-eating and drinking and underexercising and sleeping. Routine pet massage should go hand-in-hand with good nutrition and sufficient exercise, and in Chapter 9 you will find guidelines for general health maintenance for your cat.

In time, and after many experiences using massage as both a preventive health measure and a healing technique, I have worked out the system of pet massage which is described in this book. My knowledge and skills as a veterinarian, as an animal psychologist, and as a certified massage therapist combined naturally to help me discover this holistic therapy and the first massage system for animals.

THE HEALING TOUCH FOR CATS

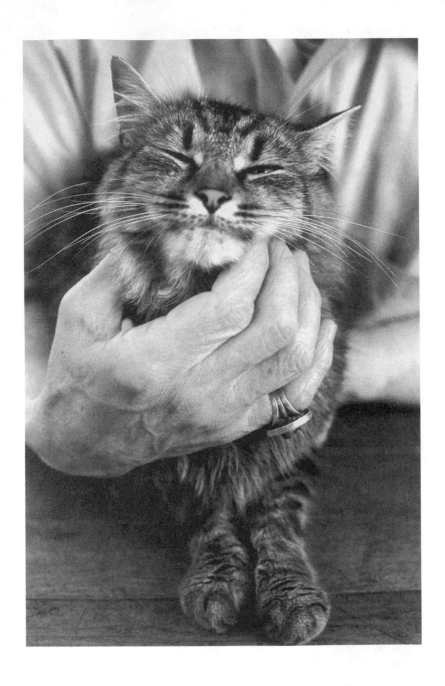

THE HEALING TOUCH

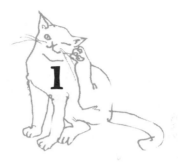

My program of massage for cats is a unique synthesis of several different massage techniques or "schools" which have been extensively researched and applied to humans. Some, like acupressure, have been used for centuries; others, like Polarity therapy and Rolfing, are more recent developments. Polarity therapy (like acupressure and Shiatsu) is based upon the principle of energy fields or currents in the body. Rolfing is a deep massage that focuses upon groups of muscles, the connective tissue between them, and postural and skeletal misalignments that can result from a maldistribution of muscle tone.

It is ironic that massage has never been applied to animals on any systematic or consistent basis, considering that animals suffer many human diseases and are treated with the same antibiotics, steroids, hormones, etc. In fact, animals are used in research studies to find cures for human diseases, precisely because they have similar and sometimes identical disorders, such as diabetes and glaucoma. Is it not logical, then, that many of the human massage techniques developed over the centuries are applicable to animals? Why has no one thought of developing a system of massage suitable for our companion animals? Perhaps it is because the massage experience is so subjective.

How will we know if the massage is of benefit to an animal if it cannot respond vocally? The answer is clear to anyone who has had a pet for even a short period of time. Once an animal is a member of your household, you certainly can tell whether it is feeling contentment, pleasure, pain, rage, depression, guilt, jealousy, or whatever.

The cats in my life have always enjoyed extensive massage from me (and from my wife and children). One of my cats, Sam, became afflicted out of the blue with feline cystitis, which resulted in a blockage of his urinary tract, painful straining, and muscular spasms in the pelvic and lower back muscles. I combined massage with standard treatment for this disorder, and he quickly recovered.

When Sam subsequently had a bout of cystitis, he would solicit a massage from me, especially a massage of the muscles around the root of the tail. He'd crawl into my lap, look at me, meow, and then place himself in the usual position I put him in to massage his hind end. Coincidence? Perhaps, but why did he only do this when he was sick? And why would he come back for more if it didn't make him feel better? Ten to fifteen minutes, twice a day, of gentle, deep kneading around this region eliminated the muscular spasms and frequent straining to pass urine which occurs in this condition even when the bladder is empty.

There are always some people who suffer from what I call "mechanistic thinking." They believe that it is wrong to attribute humanlike emotions to animals. In fact, this kind of thinking is widespread among academics. I recently heard a college professor proclaim that "all anthropomorphism is unscientific," meaning that it is wrong to attribute any emotion or feeling to animals that humans have, such as pain, pleasure, hunger, or fear. With this kind of mind-set, how could he possibly believe that animals might benefit from a gentle touch or from massage therapy?

And yet other scientists have shown through studies that deprivation of affection is as damaging to an animal (or a person) as being deprived of an essential dietary nutrient. Young cats and dogs (and other animals), like human infants, can waste away when separated from their mothers and when they are not given affectionate contact, even though their physical needs for warmth or food are provided.

The tender, loving touch is essential for well-being and for the normal growth and development of all socially dependent animals. It would seem that their nervous systems require such stimulation either from the gentle licks of their mothers' tongues or the strokes of a caring human hand. As a seedling cannot thrive without the light of the sun, so, too, do our animal kin suffer without the energy of love. And it is through touch especially that this energy can be given and reciprocated.

Please note that I said "reciprocated." There may be added hidden benefits to giving your pet a regular massage! Researchers at the University of Pennsylvania have found that people who have suffered a coronary attack are less likely to have a relapse if they have an animal at home to pet. This is the result, they believe, of a relaxing, beneficial decrease in heart rate which occurs while a person is stroking the pet—a genuine health bonus!

I am one with Hamlet when he observed, "There are more things in heaven and earth, Horatio, then are dream't of in your philosophy." In other words, I think that there is more to the healing process than Western mechanistic medicine has yet dreamed about, as witness Norman Cousins' account of his own miraculous self-healing in his best-selling book *Anatomy of an Illness as Perceived by the Patient: Reflections on Healing and Regeneration*. The book demonstrates convincingly how a positive state of mind can help the ailing body back to health. Through massage and the laying on of hands, a healing power may be transmitted which many people have experienced and many healers have verified.

There are some people who doubt the values of massage. Usually, they are people who have not experienced massage for themselves. I, too, was a nonbeliever until I had various types of massage and body manipulations (such as Rolfing and Shiatsu) done on me. It stands to reason that as a veterinarian, trained in allopathic (standard Western) medicine, I was very skeptical about all of this "touch business" until I had begun training as a massage therapist.

One afternoon I was practicing on a fellow student who had a sore throat, and after manipulating certain areas around the student's neck and shoulders, I suddenly developed a sore throat too.

Imagination, you might think. And so did I, at first. But there was no getting away from it. The more I worked on the student, the more painful and sore my own throat became!

I couldn't believe what was happening and told my instructor. She didn't seem surprised. "Go and finish the massage," she said. "Then wash up and shake your hands to 'shed' yourself of what you have picked up, and then sit down for a while." I did what she suggested and within five minutes my sore throat was gone and my fellow student was feeling much improved. I call this "sympathetic resonance." Other healers have reported similar experiences. Some can, in fact, develop such sympathetic resonance that they can "feel-see" just where the patient is suffering pain, sometimes even without touching him. Accepting the notion of massage therapy—especially of animals—does entail breaking some cultural and conceptual taboos and barriers, but there is a reward for the courageous.

It is important to remember that massage therapy is not a panacea. One should not be tempted to try it as a home cure when a pet is sick, without first having the animal examined by a veterinarian. But provided one follows the basic rules of massage, the healing touch is generally safe and without adverse side effects.

Touch and massage can help, I believe, to reconnect us with the intuitive "wisdom of the body." This body wisdom—the connection between body-sensitivity and mind-awareness—has been almost lost to modern civilization, which separates mind from body, man from animal, and humanity from nature. We have to relearn the fact that our bodies are not machines, nor are the bodies of animals.

Albert Schweitzer, the great humanitarian and healer, said that the good doctor simply awakens "the physician within" the patient. Apparently, touch and massage have this same triggering effect.

I believe that touch is one of the greatest gifts humans can share. Possibly, it is even greater when we bestow the healing touch on our dependent animal kin!

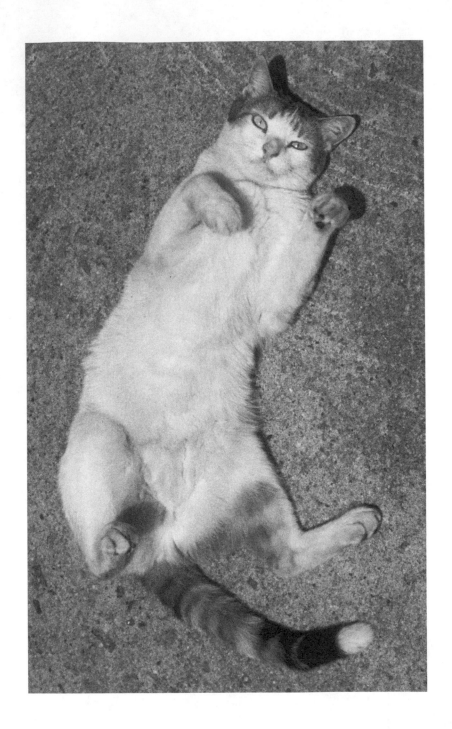

WHY CATS NEED MASSAGE

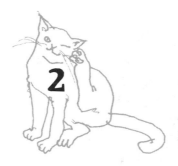

On the surface, massage may seem like a frivolous idea, but the fact is that massage has so many physical and psychological benefits for your cat that you could almost call it an essential of health care, like grooming, feeding, exercise, etc. In fact, I might go so far as to say that, for certain reasons (which I will go into later), pets benefit more from massage than human beings do.

THE PRICE OF DOMESTICATION

Skeptics might argue that since wild animals don't massage each other, it's pointless—and anthropomorphic—to believe that pets might need and enjoy a regular massage. But, in fact, animals in the wild do engage in one form of massage—social grooming. When a cat licks its offspring, that act (and you might call it superficial massage) facilitates the digestive process. Kittens weaned and separated too young will not thrive, because they don't have adequate physical contact (tender loving care) with their mothers.

Animals in the wild also play, hunt, run, and perform a full range of physical activities daily—you might say it's their form of calisthenics or natural hatha yoga. Our pets, confined indoors most of the time, lack such constant toning-up and therefore benefit from a tonifying massage. Also, domesticated animals live much longer than their wild counterparts, and many old-age problems respond well to massage therapy.

I remember one feline patient named Strawberry, an eighteen-year-old "alley" cat who had multiple health problems—arthritis, poor circulation, and kidney function—and no zest for life. Conventional veterinary treatment was helping some, but Strawberry only came back to his lively old self after his human companions put him on the right home-prepared recipes and gave him no commercial, processed cat food, as I advised, and gave him a routine massage three times a day. Once his human companions had learned the Healing Touch, Strawberry demanded it for four good years before he passed on. Massage therapy helped alleviate this aging cat's poor circulation and painful joints.

The domestic environment can also play a role in feline health and well-being. For example, I have found that cats who live only with humans more often become dull, obese, and sickly than cats whose social environment is enriched by the companionship of other affectionate, playful cats. Essentially, having two cats is a better idea than just having one. Domestic cats, who have been hand-raised and socialized early in life with humans, tend to be more dependent and infantile in their behavior than their wild counterparts. As a result, they have a greater need to be given tender, loving care. This can be in the form of random petting or it can be a systematic pleasurable stimulation from the massage system described in this book.

DIAGNOSTIC FINGERTIPS

Via regular massage, you will learn to spot when your cat needs veterinary attention much sooner than you can now with your normal "once-overs." Yes, massage actually has a diagnostic function! And the resultant early detection of illness could well save your cat much undue suffering—perhaps even his life. How many cases I recall which would have been easier for me to treat had the owners correctly spotted their pets' problems earlier. I'm thinking of Tiger, for instance, who was brought to me suffering from a fever. The owners had noticed that the cat was limping and had decided she was suffering a simple sprain that would soon heal. Except that it didn't! Had they massaged Tiger regularly, they would have felt a swelling under the skin and known that something more than a simple sprain was involved. On examining the cat, I found a deep bite wound that had become an abscess.

Sometimes it happens that a usually loving pet becomes aggressive when you accidentally touch it, hissing or clawing defensively. I have come across owners who have punished a cat for such behavior and even considered having it put down when, in fact, the poor animal had an infected ear or slipped disc that hurt terribly whenever it was touched! Once you have developed sensitive fingertips, such a tragic misinterpretation of your pet's reactions can be avoided.

AN AID TO CIRCULATION

Massage also has a therapeutic or healing function. It is extremely effective, for instance, in helping animals recover from certain injuries. A cat recovering from a sprained wrist or fractured leg will be helped greatly by appropriate massage to the afflicted limb.

How does massage help the healing process? By increasing the circulation, and by helping to reduce the build-up of fibrous tissue adhesions, which make it both difficult and painful for the animal to move. A number of illnesses respond well to massage, too, and so you will, in a sense, be assisting your vet in restoring your pet to health.

By stimulating the lymphatic as well as blood circulation, massage acts as a tonic for our old and convalescing animals, particularly those suffering from impaired heart or kidney function. As circulation is stimulated, toxins are removed from the tissues and nutrients supplied.

Most older animals suffer from other degenerative and chronic disorders which benefit from the stimulating, tonifying effects of massage. Muscular cramps, early-morning stiffness, arthritis, certain spinal disorders, and some skin conditions, for example, will improve with regular massage. Very much like their masters, pets get comfort and benefit from the reassuring and healing touch of massage.

THE BONDING TOUCH

Research has shown that physical contact for an animal who is emotionally attached to a human being is as rewarding as being given a morsel of favorite food. However, not all cats enjoy being touched. Touch-shyness, or the fear of being touched in one area of the body, such as the head or lower back, can be a sign of sickness. Or it can be the result of improper handling in early life. By "improper handling" I don't necessarily mean that the animal was abused. It's possible that the animal simply was not around people during its first few critical weeks of life—the time for developing emotional attachments. This early attachment is called "bonding."

If your cat shies away when you touch its head, for instance, that could be a sign of an ear or tooth problem. It could also indicate touch-shyness or what we sometimes call a touch phobia. How will you tell the difference? If sensitivity to touch in a certain area appears suddenly, the culprit is most likely a local infection or injury.

How do you help your cat to overcome touch-shyness if it is psychological and not physical in nature?

- Approach the animal with gentleness at all times.
  Either sit down or squat.

- Encourage the cat to approach you, touch, and sniff your extended fingers.

- Never try to touch it suddenly or lunge at it,
  even in playfulness.

- Be still and let the cat observe you, approach you,
  and rub against you.

- Speak to it softly and kindly as you try to touch it.

- Increase your touch gradually.

- Give the cat a food reward when it lets you touch it.

- It is always best to remain still and let the shy animal come to you, and food is a good motivator for many. Then later, your touch.

Touch is a potent bridge for love, and it is indeed tragic when animals lose out on both the enjoyment of being touched and the experience of reciprocating affection. Massage can help bond a kitten early in life; when continued on a regular basis, it can also help maintain the bond between cat and owner all through the animal's life.

TOUCH BENEFITS

Another important bonus from massage is that you will be accustoming your pet to being handled. This could save your cat's life some day. As a veterinarian, I can tell you how difficult and frustrating it sometimes is to deal with touch-shy animals—especially if a complicated procedure is involved. Some pets have to be tranquilized or muzzled or restrained for a simple check-up at the animal doctor's, much less a major treatment!

My mail is full of letters from people lamenting that they cannot bathe their animals, or cut their cat's claws, or even get a brush on their coats. Many an animal gives the groomer such a rough time that he has no other choice than restraint, which is traumatic, or tranquilization, which can be overdone. Once you accustom your pet to massage by yourself or other members of your family, it will be more accepting of all kinds of handling—from the vet to the barber and manicurist at the beauty salon to being placed in a crate for traveling. Being accustomed to touch will also make it easier for handlers and judges if you have an animal you wish to show. And—as a happy by-product—handling will result in a pet who is more relaxed around children and visitors. The bonuses are many.

Finally, as our lifestyles change—becoming more mechanized and removed from our own animal origins—massage becomes for each of us a substitute for certain losses. I recall the sad words of an elderly lady who lived alone in her apartment with her pet. "My cat," she told me, "is the only living thing that I have touched in twelve years."

For the elderly, giving their companion pets a regular massage is a real tonic. Also, it makes them feel specially needed, to be able to give more than just food and shelter. Even if they are less active and cannot go on long walks or romp with their pets, they can at least give them the Healing Touch.

Children, too, are quite capable of learning how to give an effective massage and derive special emotional benefits from it. My own two children, by the age of ten, had become competent masseurs of their pets and the rest of the family. As a result, I believe they are developing a unique body wisdom and awareness. And they are reasonably free of societal taboos about touch which rob so many people of satisfactory relationships.

In the same way that we benefit emotionally from being touched and having others in our lives to touch, so our pets benefit also, and it is possible that cases of depression in animals (as well as in people) can be greatly alleviated through massage. This is one of the reasons why I recommend people have two pets, since two animals living together tend to be happier and healthier than those that live alone. Also, they are less lonely and less destructive while left alone during those extended periods when the owners are out at work. Their grooming of each other is a form of massage.

I would not be ethical or professional if I left you with the thought that pet massage will solve all problems—or worse—that you can now dispense with your veterinarian and home-doctor your pet. No one medical technique or school holds all the answers. Massage can aid and abet your veterinarian's treatment and your general health routine, but it cannot and must not take the place of your vet's practiced diagnostic eye and therapeutic techniques.

You should, for instance, call your vet if your cat has a sprain and not massage it until the initial swelling has gone down. And, of

course, cats suffering from shock or some serious viral disease, such
as feline panleukopenia, should be left alone and not subjected to
deep massage, which could be an added stress, especially if the animal isn't used to massage. Also, when cats are sick, they often prefer to be alone. For some, the lightest stroking and laying on of
(healing) hands (see Chapter 8) is all they can take and probably
need, other than what the veterinarian has prescribed. The best that
you can do is keep them warm, properly hydrated, appropriately
medicated, and otherwise undisturbed. Overly fussy and concerned
owners can make things worse for sick and convalescing animals.
But as you become more experienced and attuned, you will know
when your sick pet wants to be massaged or simply held or stroked.

Massage therapy can be used as an adjunct to other treatment:

- As a stimulant to enhance postoperative recovery.

- As a catalyst for convalescence from sickness.

- As an adjunct to intensive care in cases of shock
  and severe debility.

- For diagnostic purposes (detailed in Chapters 7 and 8).

- Finally, as a form of communication that can transcend the
  physical and psychological barrier between animals and
  humans. This might best be described as "communion."

I would like to cap my arguments for massage with the most
telling one, namely that many pets learn to enjoy massage so much
that they become nuisances, soliciting massage at all times of the
day and night, unless you discipline them to a regular schedule! My

cats seem so happy and grateful for massage that sometimes I wonder if they will get to the point where they'll try to reciprocate and give me a massage. For sure, my cats groom me—a moist, if abrasive, feline equivalent. It is surprising how many pets respond when their owners are sick, becoming more attentive and sometimes grooming you more intensely than normal. For certain, they can tell when their owners are sick.

In the old days of the czars, so the story goes, one could have a trained bear walk on one's back for a couple of rubles—a stimulating Shiatsu-type massage! Not that I'm in favor of exploiting wild animals, but I'm reminded of this practice most mornings when my cats walk up and down my back to wake me up. I like to think it's because they want to give me a massage, but really, it's because they want their breakfast!

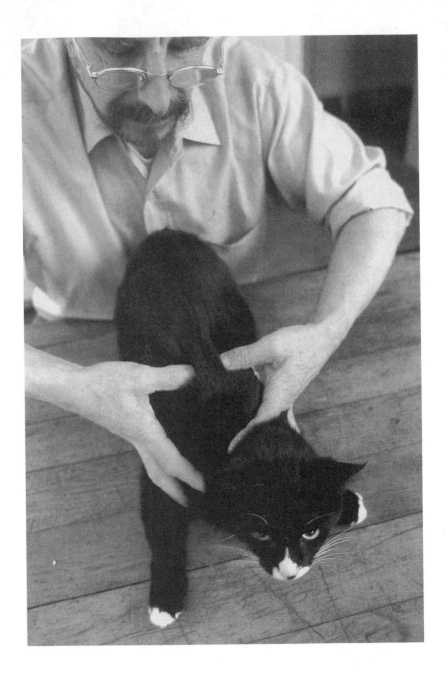

Preparing Yourself and Your Cat for Massage

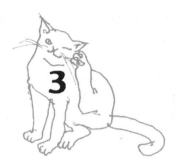

To give an effective massage, you will need, besides sensitivity, some knowledge of anatomy, and so I will give you a short and easy course on the basics in the next chapter. It is also helpful, though not essential, for you to have experienced massage yourself.

Feeling someone else's fingers beneficially manipulating your skin and muscles will make it easier for you to "feel-see" with your fingers when you massage a human friend or your animal companion. Also, the tonic effects of a massage may convince you more than any words can. You will see how touch and massage reveal the subtleties of the body and help you acquire that heightened sensitivity and intuitive wisdom which we will call body wisdom.

LEARNING BY DOING

Many people today are even more touch-shy than their pets because of society's taboos about touching. Also, being touched is anxiety-provoking, because it makes us feel more vulnerable. Since pets and children are relatively nonthreatening, and because it is socially acceptable (still) to cuddle a baby or stroke one's pet in public and in private without guilt or fear of being misjudged, people with children or pets are not as sick as they might otherwise be from touch deprivation. Society's taboos about touch have kept massage from enjoying the popularity it deserves.

If you have never experienced massage, you owe it to your body. Perhaps the motivation can be the knowledge of how much it will help you in massaging your pet.

It is not as difficult as it may seem to find a reputable masseur. First you must overcome your embarrassment at the thought of having a stranger touch your body. (I was shy and very ticklish in my first few sessions.) Then you must forget the smutty massage-parlor image that has blighted the noble and ancient art of massage therapy. You can put these unpleasant associations to rest by calling a local hospital and asking their resident physiotherapist or massage therapist for names of some state-licensed, fully qualified masseurs in your area. A local college physical education department could also give you references.

I would advise that you first go to a practitioner of standard Swedish (health-spa type) massage. As you are worked on, you will quickly learn the "feel" of the routine and experience most of the strokes and manipulations that you can later use on your pet.

The next step is to observe how the masseur gives the massage, and the best way is to watch and take notes as a friend or spouse is being worked on. Ask questions of the masseur as well as the person receiving the massage. You may even want to sign up for a course in human massage therapy which many colleges and individuals offer as evening classes or weekend workshops.

When massaging a friend, lay your fingertips or the palms of your hands very lightly on the person's skin and try to become aware of a tingling sensation. Then lift them off gently, and move them slowly over the body, about half an inch away from the body surface. Feel the temperature of the body, which is radiating heat. Eventually, you will be able to train yourself to detect areas that seem hotter or colder than normal. Painful areas, such as around a toothache, can feel quite cold, possibly because they are drawing on your energy. Such sensitivity is important for diagnostic purposes. (See Chapter 7.)

Next, see how far away you can move your hands, say from your friend's back, before the radiant energy coming from your hands can no longer be felt. If you are tired or tense, especially around the shoulders, your hands will be colder, the circulation to your hands reduced, and the energy flowing from them relatively low. If you don't feel energized, do not give a massage either to a human or animal companion, because this could fatigue you even more and lower your resistance—the motto being, "don't push the river."

THE RIGHT RELATIONSHIP

People and animals will react the same way when they lack trust in their masseurs and feel their bodies are being invaded: they will suddenly tense up. Despite themselves, many of my human clients have initially felt shy, embarrassed, or ticklish when I gave them massage. They simply had difficulty relaxing. Such reactions, of course, make it difficult to give a massage; worse, they limit its overall effectiveness.

In order to do any kind of deep-affecting massage, which involves considerable pressure, the subject must be totally relaxed. A quiet reassuring voice and a confident, firm, but gentle touch are essential ingredients; these can best be acquired through patience and experience.

It is surprising how quickly a patient, either animal or human, will learn to relax mind and body, so that he or she "flows" with the massage therapist. The subject will let you know with a groan or a protective reflex of muscle tension, or both, when you have located a particularly sensitive or painful area. Even a light touch in a hypersensitive spot, such as one of the acupressure points on the back, can be painful. But with the right trustful relationship between therapist and patient, such difficulties are quickly overcome.

Here is a checklist of a few points to keep in mind with cats that are generally hypersensitive and even afraid of light pressure manipulation:

- The secret to success is patience and perseverance. Don't give up!

- Make giving a massage a game, not a serious undertaking that must be accomplished at all costs. Forget the "even-if-it-hurts-it's-for-your-own-good" attitude.

- Never forcibly restrain the animal.

- Stroke and reassure, tickle the animal on the tummy, behind the ear, or wherever your pet especially likes to be fondled. Then follow with a few massage strokes and manipulations to the back and legs, followed by more fondling.

- Don't try to give a full massage sequence right off. The beneficial effects of even a couple of minutes' fondling and a few massage strokes and squeezes will be felt by your cat, and it will be more receptive next time and for a longer time. (It will not, however, if you use force.)

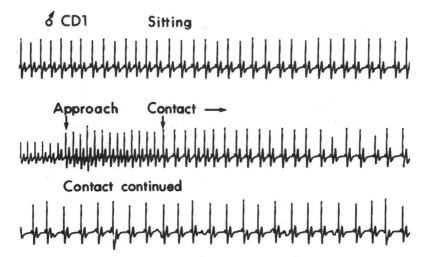

The potent effect of touch: Heartbeats in a dog (recorded with a bioteleme-ter) show how petting, stroking, grooming, etc., slows the heart to a slower rate than when sitting and during contact. Cats being approached and con-tacted by a familiar person show a similar change in heartbeat rates.

THE RIGHT MIND-SET

In preparing to massage either your pet or a friend, it is helpful to put yourself in the right state of mind first, because the wrong mind-set can do more harm than good. It is surprising to what degree the masseur's state of mind influences the quality and effectiveness of the healing touch.

Several years ago a student of mine was very eager to give me a massage in order to prove how skilled he was. After many weeks of evading him because I was leery about his mind-set, I gave in and allowed him to work on my back, which had been giving me some trouble. The next day, and for another three or four days, I could hardly move. He had put my entire back into a state of very painful imbalance, and I felt quite exhausted.

Later, I checked out how he felt, and he told me that he felt "high, energized, even lightheaded" for a day or so after he had done me in. Perhaps he had taken all my energy instead of giving me his!

Whatever the reason for our very different reactions, the young man's state of mind was, I am positive, primarily responsible for my unpleasant condition. What a contrast to my experience with the student whose sore throat I was able to help, picking up the symptoms myself in the process! Perhaps, as recent research has shown, such sympathetic resonance is linked with the fact that when a person is massaging or stroking his pet, not only the pet's heart rate decreases, but also the person's. We certainly don't need more reasons for owning and loving pets, but this research surely provides more motivation.

Some additional principles in giving massage therapy to an animal worth considering:

- Massage limbs close to where the limb joins the body, and move slowly down the limb to the paws.

- A fast and strong massage rate stimulates while a slow rate and constant rhythm sedates.

- It is better to give short 10-15 minute massage treatments frequently—four or five times a day for therapeutic purposes, once or twice for routine maintenance—than one long massage session every few days.

- To help the animal relax at the beginning of a treatment session begin with light, slow strokes (called effleurage) along the muscles and direction of the fur before going deeper and applying kneading (petrissage) and friction or deep cross-muscle fiber massage.

- Remember, massage improves blood and lymph circulation in the areas being massaged, and can enhance tissue metabolism and healing processes.

- Do not give massage to an animal with a fever, or around an infected area, or in a limb where there may be a circulatory disorder due to thrombosis, since this may cause the spread of infection or more blood clots (emboli) to develop.

- Massage causes relaxation of voluntary muscles, which is extremely beneficial in overworked muscle groups, as when an animal is lame in one foreleg and the muscles in the opposite leg get stiff and sore from taking over.

- Strained or injured muscles heal faster when massage is applied, and the development of fibrosis and adhesions between adjacent muscle fibers can be prevented or broken down by repeated treatments.

- Deep, gentle abdominal massage helps convalescent animals' digestive processes and helps relieve flatulence and constipation.

- There is some scientific evidence that massage therapy may increase beta-endorphins (natural body opiates) in the circulation and tissues; this increase is associated with relaxation, relief from pain, and a general feeling of well-being in human recipients.

- Coupling therapeutic massage with alternate cold (ice) and hot packs on an injured limb can help reduce pain and inflammation and facilitate the healing process. Ointments like Ben Gay and Tiger Balm and similar products that are used to relieve muscle and joint pain in humans should not be used on animals because they are too intense and irritating. Gentle essential oils from plants such as lavender and oregano, diluted in almond or olive oil, are preferable. These can be applied to the paws and ears and will quickly be absorbed into the animal's system.

The right mind-set is as important in massaging a pet as a person. We know that patients do better when they believe in their doctor and the treatment she prescribes. It is also true that when a doctor has a positive attitude and believes in the treatment she's prescribing, she is likely to facilitate the healing process via the placebo effect.

Triggering the natural healing processes within the body—whether by "drugless" drugs, talk, or massage—is called the "placebo effect." When Albert Schweitzer said that a good doctor simply awakens the "physician within," he was describing just this placebo effect. The great healer pointed out that witch doctors were effective with herbs and potions and rituals because their patients' minds were accessible to them.

A doctor who is hesitant, lacks confidence, and has low self-esteem and the wrong mind-set is not going to impress the patient. The same holds true for the massage therapist. Although this may sound very mystical, it really isn't, once it's experienced.

How, you might ask, can the placebo effect possibly work on a cat, or how can a cat believe in the healer or in the treatment prescribed? How, also, can we possibly know that giving an animal massage therapy is of any use?

Recent research has revealed that animals, like humans, produce natural opiate substances called endorphins and enkephalins, which may be involved in the healing process, along with another group of newly found substances called prostaglandins. These substances (and other hormones in the body, such as adrenaline, noradrenaline, and corticosteroids) are associated with reactions to physical and psychological stress and adaptation to stress.

Human experience confirms the potency of these natural opiates. The great African explorer David Livingstone was once attacked by a lion. When he was miraculously rescued, he related that after the initial attack he felt no pain while he was being severely mauled! The placebo effect most likely involves the production of some of these natural opiate substances within the body. Since we find similar substances in animals and humans, then, most likely, animals have very similar healing mechanisms (or physicians within).

Also, researchers have found that the beneficial effects of acupuncture in relieving pain may be, in part, due to the release of natural body opiates (enkephalins and endorphins) when certain points on the body are stimulated. The same euphoria, analgesia, and relaxation also occur following a good general massage that coincidentally stimulates some of the acupoints along certain meridians.

THE PLACEBO EFFECT

The presence of the healer is part of the placebo, or healing, process. Talking to an animal in a quiet, gentle voice has a very similar effect to comforting, petting, or gentle, rhythmic massage. Researchers have shown that the effect of petting is quite profound, the cardinal signs being a dramatic decrease in heart rate and a general relaxation in muscle tension. The change in heart rate is an indication that the parasympathetic nervous system is being stimulated.

There is an unconscious so-called autonomic nervous system which controls most of the vital functions of the body. It consists of two complementary parts—one being the parasympathetic system which, for example, slows the heart, and the other being the sympathetic nervous system which speeds up the heart.

The sympathetic system influences fright, fear, and flight reactions, and the parasympathetic system helps in recovery from such reactions. This dual balancing system brings about body equilibrium or what is known as homeostasis.

Chronic stress can lead to psychosomatic disturbances in animals as well as in people and cause gastric ulcers, palpitations, high blood pressure, ulcerative colitis, and increased susceptibility to certain diseases, including cancer. What massage, soft speech, and a belief in one's treatment can do is to help restore balance by stimulating the parasympathetic nervous system. This system is the damper or brake that modulates the sympathetic nervous system. This is a very simplified account of extremely complex biochemical and neurophysiological processes.

The healer, by influencing the mind of the patient, together with direct effects on the body (via drugs, massage, etc.) activates the physician within, restoring balance (homeostasis). An animal that is emotionally attached to the healer, therefore, is likely to benefit more than if it were not attached or were being treated by a stranger. This is why massage therapy holds such great potential for pet owners; its effectiveness is enhanced by the close emotional bond between pet and owner.

My Abyssinian cat Sam would let me handle him in any way. He would solicit my attention and "ask" for massage whenever he was sick. But if someone unknown to him were to lay hands on him, the stranger might be bitten. It's a question of trust. Like a young veterinarian, you have to learn the right "kennel-side" manner to win the trust of animals. Perhaps this attitude was part of the power of St. Francis of Assisi.

In sum, I believe that the placebo effect, or the awakening of the "physician within," is a product of the mental/emotional connection between healer and patient, and since animals develop strong emotional ties with their owners, there is every logical reason to believe that beneficial effects are possible. The benefit is greater, as has been proven repeatedly, if the patient believes in the healer. As you become more confident, experienced, and sensitive in giving massage to your cat, your effectiveness will be enhanced.

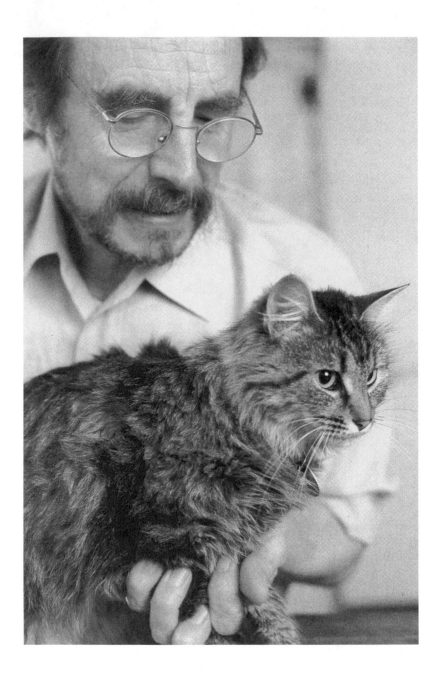

A Mini-course in Anatomy

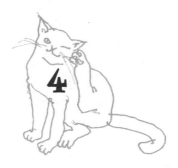

You will find it much easier to develop healing massage skills and the ability to "feel-see" while giving your pet a massage if you learn some of the basic facts about the structure and functions of the body as well as the general location of the major bones, organs, and muscles. The following modified notes from my own human massage therapy training should be very useful because basic human anatomy and physiology are the same as those of the cat. This will make your cat's anatomy easier to understand and less confusing than if I used my notes from veterinary school, which are unnecessarily detailed. You will find the basic anatomy drawings for the skeletal and muscular systems of cats and also of the location of the internal organs, on pages 34, 35, 38, and 49. Studying these will be most helpful, if not essential.

Of course, there is one major difference in the anatomy of humans and cats: our pets are quadrupeds, walking on all fours, and so their limbs are positioned quite differently from ours.

Note how the shoulder blade, or scapula, of the cat is located on the side of the body, while in us the two scapulas are rotated backwards and lie across our backs. We have collarbones, which are vestigial and nonfunctional in cats. Note, also, how cats are up on their toes, so to speak, so that they literally walk on their toes and fingers and have fore and hind legs like coiled springs. In contrast, we walk on our heels, as though we were partially hamstrung.

Notice, too, how the animal's chest is compressed laterally so that the thorax is flattened from the sides, while in us it is flattened from front to back. We have well-developed pectoral or chest muscles in the front, while in cats they are located between the front legs and are much smaller. We also have well-developed buttocks or gluteal muscles, while cats, partly because their pelvis is more horizontal than ours, have poorly developed gluteal muscles. By far, their most developed muscles are gastrocnemius or calf and related thigh muscles in the hind legs. These have evolved for leaping; and the back muscles, with the spinal column like a flexible whip, is an adaptation to facilitate locomotion and the capture of prey.

YOUR CAT'S BASIC ANATOMY

- ANATOMY is the study of the structures of the body.

- PHYSIOLOGY is the study of the normal functions of the organs of the body.

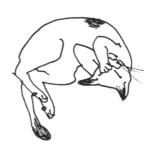

A **cell** is the smallest complete unit in the body. Groups of cells form different tissue such as:

- Skin

- Muscles

- Cartilage

- Connective tissue

- Bones

- Nerves

- Blood

- Glands

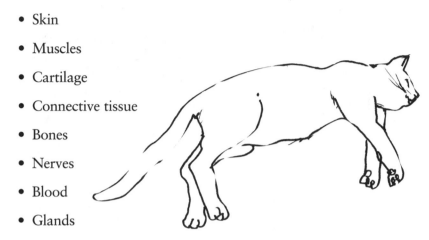

Metabolism is tissue change. It is the continuous breaking-down and building-up of cells in the body tissue, as the body takes in nutrients and casts out waste products.

Chronic means long continued. In some chronic cases, tissue change is greatly interfered with, resulting in accumulation of waste matter or toxic poisons.

THE SENSES
The five special senses and their organs are:

1. Seeing   1. Eyes

2. Smelling   2. Nose

3. Tasting   3. Tongue

4. Hearing   4. Ears (also for balance/equilibrium)

5. Feeling   5. Skin

THE BODY

The nine principal systems of the body are:

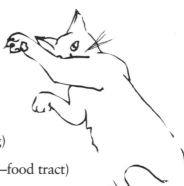

1. Skeletal (or bones)

2. Muscular

3. Nervous

4. Vascular (or circulatory)

5. Respiratory (or breathing)

6. Alimentary (or digestive—food tract)

7. Excretory (or throwing off wastes)

8. Internal Secretions (or glandular)

9. Reproductive

The **trunk** of the body is divided into:

• Thorax   • Abdomen   • Pelvis

The thorax contains **lungs, aorta, heart, esophagus.**

The abdomen contains **stomach, liver, spleen, kidneys, small intestines, colon.**

The pelvis contains the **bladder, rectum, reproductive organs.**

Skin and **fur** are a:

- protective covering of the body
- an organ of sense (feeling)
- an eliminator of waste (through sweat glands mainly on feet)
- regulator of body temperature (panting being the main way in cats)

There are two layers of skin:

1. Epidermis or outer layer

2. Dermis or true skin, containing: sweat and other glands, hair roots, capillaries, and many nerve endings

Glands are two types: duct and ductless.

Largest duct glands (with tubes)	Largest ductless glands (without tubes)
• Liver	• Spleen
• Pancreas	• Thyroid
• Kidneys	• Adrenals

Liver: Secretes bile, necessary to digestion; changes sugar to glycogen for cell use and uric acid to urea; prevents poisons from reaching the bloodstream.

Pancreas: Makes pancreatic juice necessary to digestion; secretes insulin.

Kidneys: Excrete urine, which is waste matter from the blood (the bladder is for storage of urine only).

Spleen: Forms white blood cells and helps control certain infections.

Thyroid: Regulates growth of fatty tissue, influences metabolism.

Adrenals: Help regulate blood pressure; make anti-inflammatory corticosteroids.

Organs of excretion or elimination are those that throw off wastes from the body. They are:

• Skin: Eliminates waste by perspiration.

• Lungs: give off carbon dioxide.

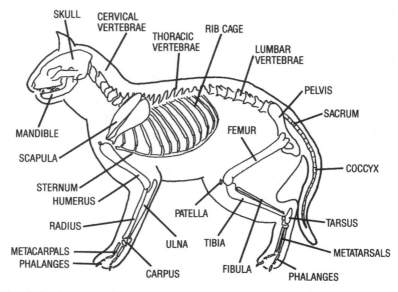

The skeletal system of the cat

- Kidneys: excrete urine, waste fluid from the blood.

- Intestines: Process undigested residue from food.

Skeleton or **bone structure** is the framework supporting the body, offering protective covering for vital organs, allowing for locomotion and providing a surface for the attachment of muscles.

Bones are made of mineral salts, mostly calcium. There are four shapes of bones:

- Long—in arms, legs, and digits

- Short—in wrist, ankle or hock, and knee

- Flat—shoulder blade, ribs, and some in head

- Irregular—vertebrae forming spine, sacrum, tail, and some skull bones

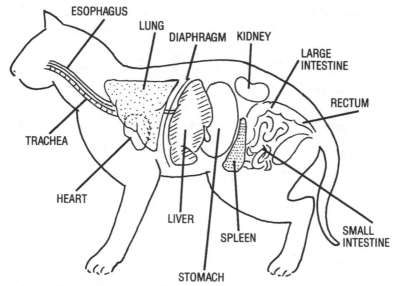

ESOPHAGUS
LUNG
DIAPHRAGM   KIDNEY
LARGE
INTESTINE
RECTUM
TRACHEA
HEART
LIVER
SPLEEN
SMALL
INTESTINE
STOMACH

Location of internal organs in the cat

Sternum is the breast bone.
Major bones are located as follows:

- Shoulder—the scapula (shoulder blade).

- Foreleg includes the humerus, radius, and ulna.

- In the forepaws are the phalanges (or toes), the long metacarpal bones, and the wrist or carpal bones.

- The bones of the spine are the cervical vertebrae, the thoracic or dorsal vertebrae, the lumbar, sacral, and coccygeal or tail vertebrae.

- The ilium is a part of the hip bone or pelvis.

- Hind leg includes the femur, tibia, and fibula, and the

kneecap, or patella. In the hind paws are the phalanges (toes), the long metatarsal bones, and the tarsal, hock, or ankle bones.

The **alimentary canal** or digestive system extends from the mouth to the anus, and parts of the alimentary canal, in order, are:

- Mouth
- Pharynx
- Esophagus (or gullet)
- Stomach
- Pyloric valve
- Small intestines (composed of duodenum, jejunum, ileum)
- Colon (or large intestine)
- Rectum
- Anus

Most of the digestion takes place in the stomach and small intestines.

The wavelike process in the colon, called peristalsis, propels the contents of the colon on toward the anus. This can sometimes be felt or seen, especially in a nervous or sick animal.

The **nervous system** coordinates the workings of all parts of the body. It is the communication system between the brain and all other parts. The nervous system regulates all movements of the body, both voluntary and involuntary. It controls digestion, elimination, and glandular action. It regulates the senses, will power, and respiration.

The two parts of the nervous system are:

- Cerebro-spinal
- Autonomic

The **cerebro-spinal** or **central nervous system** includes the brain, spinal cord, and connecting nerves. This system controls voluntary muscles and sensations. Motor impulses are carried by motor nerves to muscles when one wills to move a muscle, or from a sensory reaction such as touching something hot.

Three important parts of the brain are:

1. Cerebrum—largest part, containing centers of intelligence, will, memory, and all special senses

2. Cerebellum—lower back portion; preserves equilibrium or body balance

3. Medulla oblongata—in the back of the skull, contains automatic centers, such as respiration, sweat, vomiting, etc.

The **spinal cord** is like a telephone cable, each nerve insulated from the other. This group of nerves runs from the brain down through the spinal column, branching off between each vertebra in the spine, going to every part of the body.

The **autonomic nervous system** parallels the nerves of the cerebro-spinal system throughout the body. It aids respiration, circulation, digestion, elimination, glands, and certain vital organs. It works automatically and is so sensitive that the body is affected by fear, pleasure, shock, stress, and sickness.

Both nervous systems are closely related.

Brachial refers to the foreleg:

• The brachial artery is the largest artery in the leg.

• The brachial vein is the largest vein in the leg.

• The brachial plexus is the largest nerve group in the leg.

The largest nerve in the body is the **sciatic nerve**, which starts at the sacral region, passing under the gluteal (buttocks) muscles, and

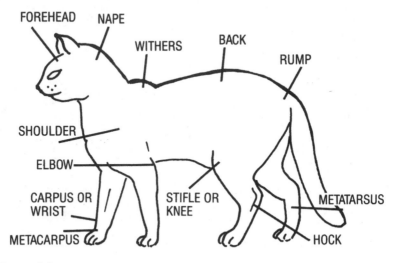

Parts of the cat

running down inside of the hind leg to the knee, where it branches into two parts, thence to the foot.

Afferent nerve impulses are those carried to the center or brain—usually sensory nerves.

Efferent nerve impulses are those carried away from the center—usually motor nerves.

A **nerve injury** will cause numbness or paralysis with lack of proper blood supply to the part of the body the nerve serves. For example, an injury to the radial nerve in the foreleg may cause the wrist and paw to hang limp with no sense of feeling in them.

Reflexes or **reflex action** refer to responses to stimulation which normally, unconsciously, serves a number of purposes. For example, if one strikes the tendon just below the kneecap, the quadriceps muscle contracts, extending the hind leg.

Joint movements are:

- Flexion—bending

- Extension—extending

- Abduction—drawing away from the middle of the body

- Adduction—drawing back to the center

- Circumduction—free movement

- Rotation—almost complete movement around

THE CIRCULATORY (VASCULAR) SYSTEM

The circulatory system controls the circulation of the blood through the body in a steady stream, by means of the heart and blood vessels, whose function it is to supply body cells with nutrient materials and carry away waste products.

The circulatory system consists of the heart, arteries, veins, capillaries, and lymphatics.

The heart is a hollow, muscular organ located in the chest cavity between the lungs and is enclosed in a sac or membrane, the pericardium. The term "cardiac" refers to the heart. The interior of the heart is divided by muscular walls into four cavities, or chambers, with four valves. The upper thin-walled cavities are the right and left auricle, and the lower thick-walled chambers are the right and left ventricles. The valves allow the blood to flow in only one direction, either forward or backward, through the eight large blood vessels which are connected with the heart. There is no connection between the left and right side of the heart. In a normal adult cat the heart beats about 110–180 beats per minute.

The venous blood returning to the heart comes into the right auricle from the two largest veins in the body. These large veins are the anterior vena cava and the posterior vena cava. When the right auricle is filled with venous blood, the tricuspid valve opens into the right ventricle which is on the same side of the heart directly below it. From the right ventricle the venous blood is carried by the pulmonary artery to the lungs. At the lungs the blood gives up its waste as carbon dioxide gas, and the red blood corpuscles pick up oxygen from the air.

Having been purified in the lungs, the blood now passes through the pulmonary veins into the left auricle. When the left auricle is filled with arterial blood, the bicuspid valve opens into the left ventricle, which is on the same side of the heart, directly below the left auricle.

From there the arterial blood passes out into the aorta, then through its many branches, on into the capillaries to nourish the tissue, returning to the heart again through the veins. The blood circulation takes less than one minute to make the complete round.

Please note this exception to the rule: the venous blood being pumped from the heart to the lungs goes through the pulmonary arteries. Likewise, the arterial blood from the lungs to the heart passes through the pulmonary veins.

The general rule on arteries and veins is: Arteries are the blood vessels (tubes) carrying purified blood away from the heart to all parts of the body. This blood is also referred to as arterial blood. Veins carry impure blood back to the heart. The blood is sometimes called venous blood. The exception to the rule is given above.

Capillaries are the hair-like tubes connecting arteries and veins all over the body.

Portal System refers to the blood vessels around the liver.

Blood contains:

- Plasma or yellowish fluid

- Red blood corpuscles which carry oxygen

- White blood corpuscles, which fight and resist infection, and also carry nourishment to the tissue.

Production of blood is aided by bone marrow, the liver, and the spleen. The blood-vessel walls are porous, allowing food or nourishment to be absorbed by the tissue. Also, waste from many parts seep through the lymph and into the blood to be carried away.

Lymph is similar to blood without red blood cells, and it is more fluid. The lymphatic vessels are an independent set of vessels which aid the veins. Lymph help nourish cells in every tissue. The white blood cells in the lymph help fight and resist infection through the body. Lymph capillaries unite to form larger lymphatics. The two largest ducts in this system are:

- Thoracic duct • Right lymphatic duct

Lymph nodes, small glands along the lymphatics, also help prevent the spread of infections. White cells are made in the spleen and, by division in the lymphatics, multiply themselves.

THE RESPIRATORY SYSTEM
The Respiratory System includes:

- Nose
- Mouth
- Lungs
- Pharynx
- Windpipe or trachea
- Bronchial tubes

The **larynx** is the organ of voice.

The **lungs** are somewhat elastic and filled with sacs like a sponge. The blood takes on oxygen in the lungs and gives off carbon dioxide (or waste).

The **diaphragm** is a large, flat, muscular organ that separates the thoracic and abdominal cavities. Its action aids inhalation, expiration, and defecation.

THE MUSCULAR SYSTEM

Muscles consist of long fibrous tissue with stretching ability. Muscles move every part of the body and make up internal organs. There are about 600 muscles in the body. There are two classes of muscles: voluntary and involuntary.

- Voluntary muscles are controlled by will.

- Involuntary muscles are not under control of will, such as in the heart and colon.

Tendons are the ends of muscles that attach to the bone.

A **ligament** is a band of fiber connecting bones.

Cartilage is thin flat fiber between the vertebrae and in joints, and acts as a cushion between the bones.

Synovial fluid lubricates around cartilage tissue.

Muscle tone means not flabby.

Fatigue is accumulation of waste, due to lack of sufficient nourishment or poor elimination.

By **origin** and **insertion** of muscles, we refer to both ends of the muscles where they are attached to bones.

Action of a muscle is what it does:

Flexor—bends

Extensor—straightens out

Rotator—permits turning

Muscles can also be adductors and abductors.

For details about the names and locations of the major skeletal muscles, see the diagram on page 49. Also, refer to the text in Chapters 7 and 8.

Major muscles are:

- Big neck muscle—sternocephalicus (from sternum to the mastoid process of the temporal bone)
  Action: Moves head toward shoulder or chest

- Upper back muscle—trapezius (from occipital bone, down the spine, including the 12th dorsal vertebra to the scapula)
  Action: Lifts the shoulders

- Back muscles—latissimus dorsi (from last six dorsal vertebrae down the spine, to the humerus)
  Action: Bends foreleg back or down and draws trunk forward when the limb is advanced

- Longissimus dorsi (in the lower back region)
  Action: Extends and flexes the spine

- Inside foreleg muscles—pectorals (from sternum and upper ribs to humerus)
  Action: Moves foreleg across chest

- Between the ribs—intercostals (two muscles in each space, connecting the ribs)
  Action: Help the ribs protect the chest and aid respiration

- Between the chest and abdomen—diaphragm
  Action: Helps respiration (breathing)

- Shoulder muscle—deltoid (from foreleg, scapula to humerus)
  Action: Advances and rotates the foreleg

- Foreleg muscles—biceps (from scapula to radius)
  Action: Bends the elbow and supinates the paw

- Triceps
  (from scapula and humerus to ulna)
  Action: Extends the foreleg

- Forearm muscles—(from humerus to
  wrist and digits) Pronators: turn
  paw down
  Supinators: turn paw up
  Flexors: bend wrist and digits
  Extensors: extend wrist and digits

- Buttocks muscles—3 layers of gluteal
  muscles (from ilium, sacrum, and
  coccyx to femur)
  Action: Move the thigh

- Hind-leg muscle—quadriceps femoris
  (from ilium and femur to patella)
  Action: Extends the leg

- Biceps femoris (from hip bone and femur to tibia and patella)
  Action: Extends hip and bends the knee

- Calf muscle—gastrocnemius (from femur to heel bone)
  Action: Extends the foot and flexes leg. Its tendon (of Achilles
  or the hamstring) attaches to the heel bone

- The major muscles of the head are the masseter and the
  temporal muscles.

SUMMARY

The **skeletal system** consists of the bones of the body. Their main function is support.

The **muscular system** consists of voluntary and involuntary muscles. Their main function is to contract and cause motion.

The **digestive system** consists of the digestive canal and accessory glands, the function of which is to receive, digest, and absorb food to nourish all the structures of the body.

The **circulatory system** consists of the heart, blood vessels and blood, lymphatics and lymph. Its main function is to distribute body fluids to all the cells, take food to the cells, and remove wastes.

The **nervous system** consists of the central or cerebrospinal nervous system, which controls the voluntary muscles and all sensation, and then the autonomic nervous system, which controls all the involuntary muscles. The function of these two branches of the nervous system is to control and insure coordination in the working of all the systems of the body.

The **respiratory system** consists of the nose, larynx, trachea, bronchi, and lungs. Its function is to provide oxygen to the bloodstream and to remove wastes in the form of carbon dioxide.

The **excretory system** consists of the bowels, kidneys, skin, and lungs. Its function is to eliminate all the waste products of the body.

These systems are integrated with the ENDOCRINE (including the reproductive) and IMMUNE SYSTEMS and together maintain homeostasis—the regulation and balance of all physiological processes and bodily functions.

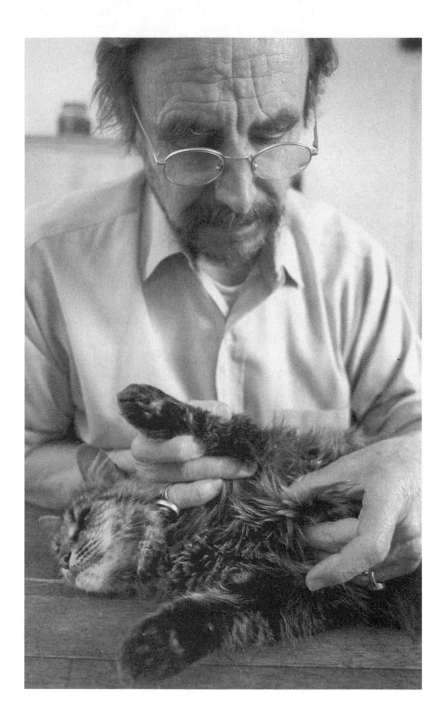

UNDERSTANDING YOUR CAT'S BODY LANGUAGE

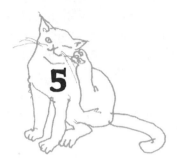

It is important to recognize your cat's body-surface subtleties, because touching areas during stroking or massage can evoke some surprising behavioral responses! As the animal begins to relax, for instance, feelings of sexual arousal are quite common. This behavior will disappear quickly as the massage sequence proceeds. Fleeting sensations of sexual arousal may also be experienced by the person giving the massage. This, too, is quite natural, since sexual or libidinal energy is one manifestation of the life force that is thought to be the energy transmitted during massage.

At first, your cat may resist certain massage procedures. Don't be surprised; just be patient and persevere. As I pointed out, it takes weeks for many people to get used to being touched in certain places because they are ticklish or shy, or they may find some areas too painful to take much manipulation and pressure.

I keep my mind focused on the rhythm of my own breathing and on the patient's. Any change in the depth or frequency of the patient's breathing can mean that pain is being experienced, that the animal is afraid, tense, relaxing, or even going to sleep. I also focus my attention as continuously as possible on the image of energy flowing from me, through my hands, and into the patient.

Sometimes an animal or person may feel this energy suddenly and react as though jolted. Sudden tensing can also mean that the pressure you are applying is too hard or the patient is afraid of what you are doing. Or it can mean that you have found a significant tender spot that is of diagnostic value (see Chapter 7) or one requiring special handling due to a local injury or a referred pain from some other body region. For example, pain in the lower back region in cats is often associated with kidney disease. So besides concentrating upon your own and your cat's breathing and upon the image of the healing energy flowing through your hands, your mind must be open and your senses attuned to the slightest feedback you can detect from the animal.

Certainly, your cat will let you know if you are pressing or manipulating too hard, and you can make appropriate adjustments after words of apology and reassurance—just as with a human being. Just like people, some animals prefer deeper, harder, or softer pressure than others. You will find an animal's tolerance by beginning slowly and gently, thereby helping it to relax and "open up" its body. Then, gradually, you will increase the strength of the massage until you can feel deeply into the muscular and connective tissue without causing the animal to tense or try to get up and away from you.

Personally, I find receiving a superficial massage quite unsatisfying. I feel it's a waste of time if the masseur just makes a few surface manipulations of the superficial musculature and neg-

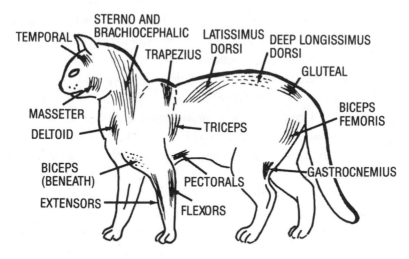

TEMPORAL

STERNO AND
BRACHIOCEPHALIC

TRAPEZIUS

LATISSIMUS
DORSI

DEEP LONGISSIMUS
DORSI

GLUTEAL

MASSETER

DELTOID

TRICEPS

BICEPS
FEMORIS

BICEPS
(BENEATH)

EXTENSORS

PECTORALS

FLEXORS

GASTROCNEMIUS

Location of major muscles in the cat

lects the deeper musculature. For this reason, I consider it essential that you know the location of the major muscle groups that you will be massaging. (See above.) It's a good idea to palpate and explore where these various muscles are located on your pet with the muscle chart in front of you. It's also essential that you know the animal's skeletal structure, how its limbs move and joints flex, extend and rotate, because several of the massage procedures involve moving the animal's appendages, and they do not move the same way as our limbs do.

There are also a number of key points on the surface of the animal's body that are of diagnostic and therapeutic value, which you will also want to learn. It is harder to find these points on animals than on humans because fur acts as an insulator, but if the fur is not too thick, you should be able to feel your pet quite easily. The body temperature of cats is two to three degrees Fahrenheit higher than ours, which does help in diagnosis. Cold areas of skin surface can, for example, indicate that the animal is in shock, is experiencing localized pain, or has a metabolic problem, such as an underactive thyroid gland, while a warmer than normal area could mean that there is local inflammation, such as a bite wound.

Unfortunately, one cannot see such things as blotching, pallor, or flushing of the skin during massage of a furry pet as one can on a human being, because these can be useful diagnostic signs. I have seen, for example, a person's face flush with color and indeed look more alive than ever, after deep massage around the neck and shoulders has released a block. Such sudden changes in energy flow or circulation can be accompanied by fine tremors especially down the arms and legs of a person. You may occasionally see similar tremors while massaging your cat. Wilhelm Reich described this as a release of "orgone," energy which occurs when a block (a tense segment of the body such as the shoulders or lower back) is removed with effective massage therapy.

PSYCHOLOGICAL ORIGINS

There are certain body regions in cats that have special social or psychological associations. Touching the abdomen of a cat that is relaxed and lying on its side can trigger a defensive reflex so that the cat bites and claws. This is very common. Similarly, some cats resent being touched near the base of the tail. Grasping a cat at the back of the neck has an immobilizing effect. This probably relates to the fact that the tomcat immobilizes the female prior to intercourse by biting her at the back of the neck. Also, the mother cat carries her kitten (which remains immobile) by this kind of neck bite. Holding a cat by the scruff of the neck does have a pacifying effect.

People, too, have their "shy spots" and become either ticklish or irritable when touched, for example, behind the shoulder blades or on the side beneath the armpits or waist. It may simply relate to having been tickled in childhood.

Female cats in heat may raise their hind end and present themselves sexually when the skin at the base of the tail is touched. This is quite natural. Kittens will often attempt to engage in playful fighting with you while they are being massaged. That's why it's a good idea to massage young animals after they have played and when they are tired and ready for a nap. (This holds true for infants as well: the best time is after its bath and just before bed.)

Many people go into a semi-hypnotic, trancelike state when they are having their hair brushed or scalps fingered or massaged. The human scalp, in my opinion, is a specially developed area of the

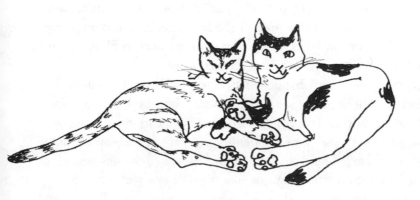

body, evolved not for keeping the brain insulated (a thick skull will do fine), but for social grooming. The extensive nerve supply to the base of each hair, which makes each hair sensitive to the slightest pressure, is the reason why the scalp is exquisitely sensitive to another's touch. In addition, the scalp is loose and thus helps protect the skull from blows, because the skin slides easily and deflects the blow. Similarly, cats' loose skins help them not only to deflect the blows of adversaries, larger creatures, and automobiles, but make it possible for them to twist around when caught and still bite defensively and wriggle free.

SMELLS AND CLUES

I have found that people's scalps smell different, so in addition to being a "grooming organ," the human scalp may also be a scent organ that may facilitate individual recognition and possibly other social behavior affected by internal hormones. Similarly, cats have organs used for social grooming and produce scent for individual recognition. Cats have scent glands along the tail, under the chin, corners of the lips and temples, just in front of the ears. Being rubbed under the chin or side of the face puts cats into an almost trancelike state, and they will return your pressure, rubbing against your hand and anointing you with their odor.

Kittens have a very distinctive "fresh-baked bread" smell on their breaths. Evolutionarily speaking, this may be an imprinting stimulus for the mother. Use your nose as best you can when massaging your pet. Your nose can help identify a variety of problems ranging from the metallic, fetid smell of an infected ear to the sickly smell of a cat with cancer, and the urine-like smell of one with uremia.

While being massaged or stroked, cats may start flexing and extending their forelegs, "kneading" with their forepaws, and salivating; they may even attempt to nurse. This is quite natural, even in old cats, who enjoy "regressing" and behaving like nursing kittens. Such reactions are often more intense in cats that have been weaned early or bottle-raised.

You may wonder of what use your cat's whiskers are. They help protect the eyes when the animal is going through dense cover. A flick on any whisker reflexively triggers the eyelids to close, and this blink reflex helps protect the eye from being poked. The whiskers, or vibrissae, which are extremely sensitive to pressure, can also tell the animal which way the wind is blowing and when it changes—important cues for a cat scenting its prey or avoiding being hunted.

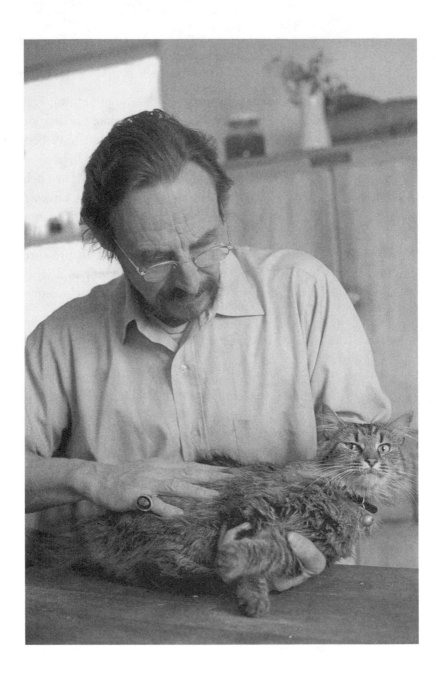

THE MASSAGE ROUTINE

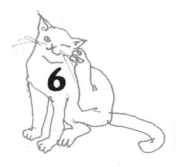

In this chapter I will offer a basic routine massage sequence that you can give to your cat every day if you wish, or at least once a week. This massage system forms the basis for therapeutic massage, described in Chapter 8. As you develop this system and acquire the essential techniques and "feel," you will also be able to apply what you have learned for diagnostic massage, as outlined in Chapter 7.

But before I outline the massage sequence itself, which goes systematically from one part of the animal's body to another in a flowing, integrated pattern, I will describe the various massage strokes that are used in the basic routine. You may need to refer to them at first. But in time, the terms will be instantly recognizable.

You may wish first to have a professional massage therapist work on you to get a "feel" for massage. Or you may ask to be allowed to observe the therapist working on another patient. And then you may wish to practice what you've learned on a friend before going on to your feline companions.

THE GENERAL MASSAGE SEQUENCE

This sequence, which you can vary to suit yourself and your pet once you have mastered the routine, consists of the following steps, which in total should take about twenty minutes to complete.

Step One: The relaxation stage makes you and the animal calm and receptive.

Step Two: Massage of the back, beginning at the nape of the neck and moving down to the rump and sacrum.

Step Three: Massage of the head and neck, including the face and jaw muscles.

Step Four: Massage of the shoulder and forelegs.

Step Five: Massage of the chest and abdomen.

Step Six: The hip and hind legs are massaged.

Because of the different arrangement of muscles and tendons in these six regions of the body, different massage strokes are needed. These will now be detailed with particular reference to the various anatomical structures that you must recognize in order to give a full and effective general body massage.

Before giving a massage, remove all sharp-edged jewelry, including wristwatches and rings, and be sure that your finger- and thumbnails are not so long that they press into or scratch the animal's skin when you are massaging.

Unlike giving a massage to a human being, you do not need to use massage oil, which would ruin your cat's coat. Even if your cat's feet or nose seem dry, I do not advise putting on oil, unless your veterinarian suggests otherwise.

MASSAGE STROKES AND MANIPULATION
1. Strokes or Passes—Effleurage

These strokes are given with the flat palm and fingers, as though you were petting the animal. At first, they should be slow and very light. (Just strong enough to pull out any loose fur.) Gradually, increase the pressure of the strokes as you proceed and stroke at a rate of about 15 strokes per minute. Strokes should be directed along the fur line, down along the back, and down from shoulder to front foot, and hip to hind foot.

You can alternate hands, or stroke with one hand and keep the other lightly on the animal's flank or head.

2. Fingertip Massage

With two or three fingers extended and kept close together, rub in a circular pattern the underlying muscles. Do not lose contact with the skin as you make small circular movements: the skin will slide easily so you can work on quite a large surface of muscles and tissue beneath. Increase the pressure as you feel the animal relax its muscles.

If you are right-handed, work with the fingers of your right hand and keep the animal quiet and down by applying gentle pressure to its side or head with the palm of your other hand.

Use your left hand to hold the leg by the hock or wrist when you are giving fingertip massage to the hip, thigh, shoulder, and foreleg.

A variation of this is vibratory massage, which entails keeping two or three fingers together in one place and shaking your wrist without taking the fingers off the skin; pressure should increase as you vibrate.

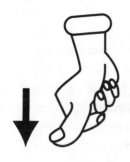

3. Acupressure

The thumbs are used for applying acupressure, except for very small cats when you use the tip of the index finger. If the animal is lying on one side, you can work with the thumb of your right hand, applying increasing pressure with the ball of your thumb to the various acupressure, or ki, points shown on page 105.

Do not make circular movements as in the fingertip massage. Simply press straight down "into" the animal as though you were pushing right through its body. Five seconds of pressure on each point is sufficient. Press as hard as the animal will allow before its relaxed muscles tense protectively. (For points that seem extremely sensitive, go carefully and refer to the next chapter on diagnostic massage.)

When giving acupressure to the limbs, hold the limb in the left hand and press down vertically onto the point with the ball of your thumb. For the back, with the animal lying on one side, make the angle in which you press go straight into the point on the back between the vertebrae as though your thumb has to come out in line, parallel with the animal's legs.

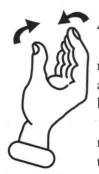

4. Deep Massage—Petrissage

This technique is analogous to kneading and rolling dough. The skin is lifted, kneaded, pulled, and rolled between fingers and thumb along the back, flank, and chest.

For the shoulder, thigh, and limbs, the deeper muscles and tendons can be kneaded between the thumb and fingers of the right hand with the left hand holding the limb and occasionally flexing and extending it (by alternately pulling and pushing the limb).

The kneading movements should be slow and rhythmic and pull across the lie of the muscle fibers and tendons for maximum benefit. Petrissage involves not direct pressure so much as actually feeling, picking up, and squeezing relaxed groups of muscles. Try this on your own calf muscle or thigh and you will quickly appreciate how good this deep manipulation feels and just how much squeezing and kneading can be given without discomfort.

5. Friction Massage

These are fast, invigorating strokes given with the balls of the first two or three fingers of one or both hands. The pressure should be sufficient to remove loose fur in quantity, but not sufficient to stop the movement from being smooth and fast.

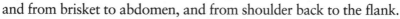

Always follow the animal's fur line from nape to rump and from shoulder or hip to foot, and from brisket to abdomen, and from shoulder back to the flank.

In contrast to slow effleurage, friction massage strokes can be at a rate of one every second, gradually increasing to twice that rate. I like to finish an invigorating massage with friction before I go to closure (the last step).

6. Closure

Extend palms and fingers, and press your hands slowly over your pet's body, barely touching it as you go. Follow the fur line from nose to tail, and sweep gently from shoulder to forepaw and rump to hind foot. Give five or ten slow passes, talking quietly to your pet, smoothing its coat and "aura" as though to seal a protective energy field around your pet that is now charged and purified after the massage that you have given. Finally, wash your hands.

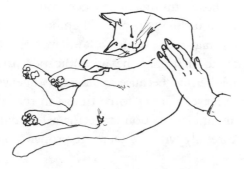

GENERAL MASSAGE ROUTINE

STEP ONE:
THE RELAXATION STAGE

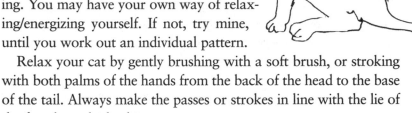

In preparing to massage a cat (or even a person), I like to close my eyes for a few moments and breathe deeply and slowly to relax and energize myself. I raise, lower, and shake my shoulders, arms, and hands, then rub my hands together to get the circulation/energy flowing. You may have your own way of relaxing/energizing yourself. If not, try mine, until you work out an individual pattern.

Relax your cat by gently brushing with a soft brush, or stroking with both palms of the hands from the back of the head to the base of the tail. Always make the passes or strokes in line with the lie of the fur along the back.

You may wish to talk quietly to the animal or have some relaxing music playing. This can help you develop a rhythm and, more important, will act as a sound barrier and mask sudden extraneous noises.

This relaxation stage preparatory to the massage session can last anywhere from 2–5 minutes. The strokes or passes should be light and slow: count slowly from 10 up to 15, beginning at the top of the cat's head and finishing when you reach 15. You'll be surprised at how quickly your pet will come to understand this is the relaxation stage and relax in anticipation. If the animal becomes agitated, that may be an indication that he is sick, injured, or apprehensive because the last massage was uncomfortable, for some reason. Don't force things in that case, but limit massage to this first relaxation stage for a few days before proceeding very carefully with the massage proper.

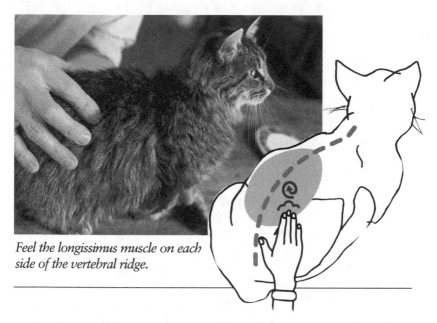

Feel the longissimus muscle on each side of the vertebral ridge.

Your pet will most likely prefer to lie on one side, though some cats like to roll over onto their backs or lie flat on their stomachs with their hind legs sticking straight out behind. While your pet is on its back, you can massage its limbs easily, but it will need to be put on one side or on its stomach or in a sitting position when you come to massage the back. (Be cautious in handling cats that are lying on their backs relaxed, until you know it's safe. Touching the abdomens of some cats can trigger a defensive aggressive reaction—biting and scratching.)

Actually, you can massage your cat in whatever position proves most comfortable. Since most animals like to lie on one side, the massage routine will be described for an animal lying on one side.

To turn your cat over, simply hold its forepaws in one hand and its hind feet in the other and, as you extend the legs, roll the animal onto its back and then over onto its side.

THE MASSAGE RITUAL

Time and patience are needed to get your pet used to the idea of being gently massaged. If you start off with kittens, a few minutes every day, combined with a little play and regular petting, you will habituate the animal to the routine. By the time the cat is six months old, you should be able to give it a good ten-to-twenty-minute session. Take the same approach with adult cats: patience—a little more deep contact and less reassuring petting each day. The equation is: total trust for total massage.

Talk to your pet in a quiet, reassuring voice. "Okay, time for relaxation. . . . Let's see how your back is doing. . . . Ah, yes, nice relaxed muscles . . ." Meanwhile, you are working with your fingers, first lightly stroking, then going deeper, but lightening the pressure the second your cat tenses.

Praise the animal for relaxing, and eventually you will feel your energies flowing together. It's almost like playing a harp or other musical instrument. Just don't pull the strings or press the keys too hard.

Choose a regular time and place for the massage, ideally not soon after the animal has been fed, or just before it expects to be fed or taken out for a walk.

Take the phone off the hook and put on some quiet music, which will help keep out sudden extraneous sounds and also condition your pet to relax.

Don't give up! Some cats never seem to accept massage because of their temperament, some past trauma, or past rearing history. Keep on trying, because you may suddenly win your pet's trust. One of my cats was quite averse to any form of sustained physical contact, but after several months we worked things out. On a number of occasions, when he was ill, he actually solicited being massaged, a clear sign that when an animal's trust is won, miracles can be accomplished.

STEP TWO: THE BACK

2.1. Fingertip Massage

First, feel where the dorsal processes or upper ridges of the vertebrae are located—right in the midline of the back, running all the way down to the animal's tail. Having located this reference point, place an index finger on each side of the ridge in the midlumbar region (see chart, page 34) and press gently. You will feel the thick, bandlike back or longissimus muscle (see chart, page 49) on each side of the vertebral ridge.

The longissimus muscle is complex, with many points of origin and termination, its functions being to flex and twist the spinal column. Stiffness of the muscle or injury to it can therefore greatly impair and restrict an animal's range of movements, and massage helps relax and tonify this important muscle group.

Begin the massage, once you have located the muscles, by making small, circular movements, with slight pressure to the muscle on each side of the spinal ridge, first in a clockwise and then a counterclockwise direction.

Start between the shoulder blades and work slowly down toward the base of the tail. Increase the pressure as much as the animal will permit. Do not lift your fingers from your cat while making these slow, circular movements down the back. Feel the skin move, and sense the muscle beneath. With repeated sessions you will quickly develop a more educated sense of touch so that you can "feel-see" how this back muscle lies in relation to the spinal ridge.

Repeat 3–4 times.

Note how the ridge consists of what feels like separate knobs: these are the dorsal or upper processes of the vertebrae. With the tip of your index finger, locate the gap between each process and follow it down until you feel the back muscle. This is a very important spot between each vertebra where bundles of nerves and ki, or acupressure, points are located.

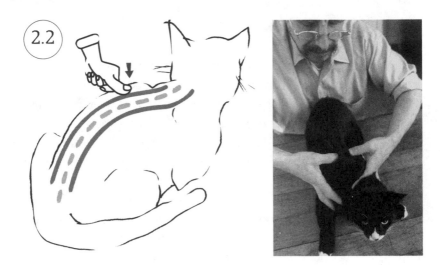

Press with the ball of your thumb on each ki point

2.2 Acupressure to the Back.

Press with the ball of your thumb (index fingertip for smaller cats) on each ki point (see chart, page 105).

Apply acupressure all the way down the back. Apply pressure gradually, because you may locate some tender spots (see Chapter 7 on diagnostic massage). You should never apply the same amount of pressure as a matter of routine: massage should not be a mechanical routine. *Feel your way.*

Ideally, the pressure should be hard. So increase pressure, making it as hard as the animal will tolerate it, without tensing its back muscles or moving to avoid contact.

The pressure should be vertical (straight down and "through" the animal) and should be maintained with no movement, for 2–3 sec-

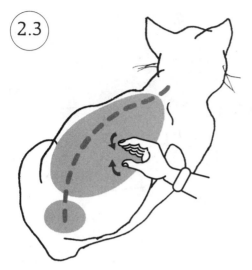

Lift, knead, pull, and roll the skin between the thumb and first two fingers.

---

onds. Breathe out as you increase the pressure, and imagine your ki or energy flowing through your fingers or thumbs into the animal.

Repeat 2–3 times.

2.3. Petrissage Massage

The third phase of the back massage is to lift, knead, pull, and roll the skin between each thumb and first two fingers. This has a general stimulating effect, and most cats enjoy it. Repeat 3–4 times.

Be careful with the skin region near the rump or base of your cat's tail. Some cats bite or scratch when this area is touched and are habitually hypersensitive in this region. Many cats are not, however, and any sudden increase in sensitivity can be of diagnostic importance. (See Chapter 7.)

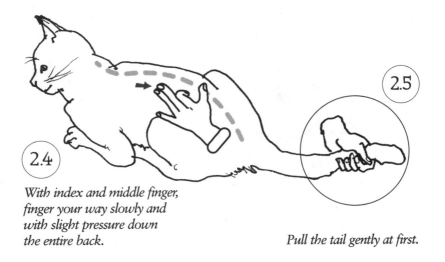

With index and middle finger, finger your way slowly and with slight pressure down the entire back.

Pull the tail gently at first.

2.4. Friction Massage

Beginning at the top of the back between the shoulder blades and with index and middle finger (plus ring-finger for larger cats), finger your way slowly and with slight pressure down the entire back. (Avoid pressing on top of the spinal ridge, because that can hurt.)

Repeat this manipulation faster and faster until you are literally sweeping your pet with long, light strokes. This is like a good brushing, but superior, because it is nonmechanical and involves direct physical contact. You may notice your pet's fur ripple. This is a natural skin contraction called the panniculus reflex. Do not do friction massage of the back too vigorously in the winter when the house is dry or with your pet lying on some synthetic material such as a nylon rug, because both of these conditions cause a charge of static electricity to build up which can give your cat (and yourself) an unpleasant shock and make massage a noxious experience. You may instead wish to give the animal a few strokes with a moist

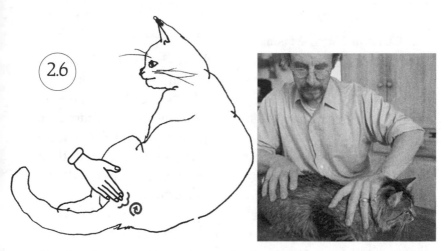

Use circular fingertip strokes in this low lumbar-sacral area for about one minute.

---

sponge first. This will help stop the buildup of an electrical charge. It's also a good way of removing loose fur.

2.5. Chiropractic-type Manipulation
(for cats accustomed to massage)

Hold the first third of the cat's tail, and pull it while holding the animal's head firmly in the other hand. (Sorry, Manx cats miss out on this one!) How hard to pull? I can't and won't tell you, because I could never be right for all pets. Let your pet teach you. This is the central law of massage—operate on the basis of feedback, and that means feel how the pet reacts.

Always pull the tail gently at first. Do it a little harder next time, and see just how far you can go. Animals, in my experience, enjoy this particular manipulation, and it is especially useful as a therapeutic procedure (see Chapter 8). One or two pulls will suffice.

2.6. Sacral or Rump Massage

Finally, massage the region around the base of your cat's tail. Use circular fingertip strokes in this low lumbar-sacral area for about one minute. Pay particular attention to the "space" between the tail and the animal's pelvis, and literally feel your way into this area. You will be able to feel the bony prominences of the pelvis and the powerful muscles around the rump: the gluteals. Massage these with fingertip strokes. Vibratory massage with fingertips is also beneficial in this area and especially for older, arthritic pets.

Cats will often raise the hind end when this region (which in humans is the buttocks and sacrum) is rubbed or stroked. It is an extremely sensitive area in most animals and even light pressure usually evokes obvious signs of pleasure. Some pets, especially cats, are hypersensitive in this area and may attempt to escape or scratch when touched. Hypersensitivity is also seen in animals that are in heat, and cats especially may present sexually, the so-called lordosis response.

Note: At this point, you can go on to massage the head and neck. If you opt for the hind legs, you should then do the abdomen, chest and forelegs, finishing up with the head and neck. Alternatively, you can proceed to the head and neck, then go to the forelegs, then chest and abdomen, finishing with the hind legs. Eventually you and your pet will work out the most compatible sequence and duration of massaging the various body regions, for a time period ranging anywhere from fifteen to thirty minutes a day.

STEP THREE: HEAD AND NECK

Feel the base of your cat's skull at the back of the neck where the head joins the first vertebra. (See chart, page 34.) There are many muscles in this region and just like people, most pets enjoy deep massage in this region. Use fingers and thumbs to give a light, circular massage at first. As the animal begins to relax, you can make

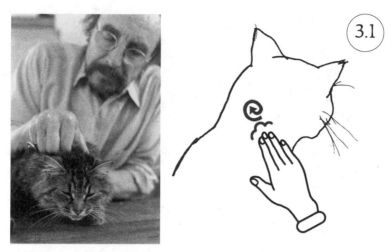

Feel the base of your cat's skull at the back of the neck where the head joins the first vertebra.

---

deeper and smaller circles. Follow the muscles forward, and feel the tendon-like attachments to the skull.

Massage in this region for one or two minutes is particularly invigorating. Cats may roll and try to rub their faces against your hands, and sometimes half close their eyes, a clear sign of pleasure.

Continue the circular finger movements under the animal's neck, first checking where the windpipe, or trachea, lies, since pressure on it will cause discomfort. You will feel a band of muscles on each side of the throat, which go up to the skull at the base of each ear. These are the sterno-mastoid and related muscles, which enable the animal to flex its head. Work in this region for at least one minute.

At the angle of the jaw, just beneath the ear, is a sensitive area very soft to the touch where salivary and lymph glands are located. Go very gently here. Swelling and pain can be a sign of sickness (see Chapter 7 for diagnostic points).

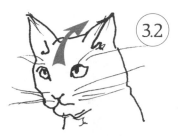

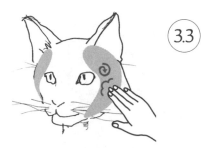

With flattened fingers, begin the head massage with gentle strokes following the lie of the fur.

Massage the temporal muscles.

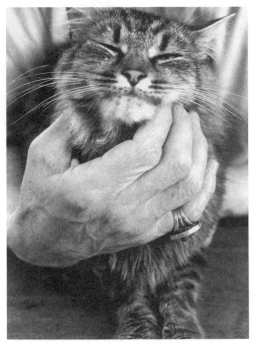

With forefinger on one side and thumb on the other, massage the jaw muscles.

Next, with flattened fingers, begin the head massage with gentle strokes following the lie of the fur from the muzzle backwards, just as you would normally pet your cat. Stroke about twelve times.

Next, apply fingertip circular massage to the major muscles of the head for one to two minutes. First, massage the powerful temporal, or temple, muscles located in front of each ear on the side of the head, and then with forefinger on

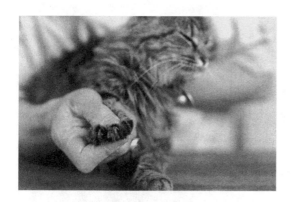

Massage, squeezing between fingers and thumb, the many muscles that lie along and between the digits or metacarpal bones.

one side and thumb on the other, massage the jaw or masseter muscles. Other superficial and deep muscles associated with the scalp region, ears, and mouth can be massaged with gentle circular movements with two or three fingertips kept close together, while the other hand supports the animal's head from beneath.

STEP FOUR: SHOULDER AND FORELEG
4.1 The Paw

Hold the leg in one hand, with the animal either lying on one side (and you working on the upper leg that is not on the massage mat or table) or in a sitting position.

Massage for at least one minute, squeezing (petrissage) between fingers and thumb, the many muscles—abductors, adductors, extensors, and flexors—that lie along and between the digits or metacarpal bones. (See charts, pages 34, 49.) Also, seize each digit and move up and down with a gentle, vibratory movement.

At the wrist or carpal region, knead across the tendons and then hold the paw and flex, extend, and inwardly rotate or supinate it to help relax and stretch the tendons around the wrist.

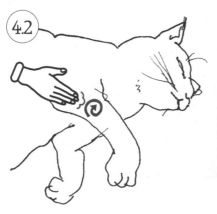

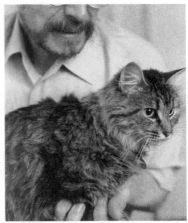

Knead across the tendons, and then hold the paw and flex, extend, and inwardly rotate it to help relax the tendons around the

Pull and push the leg alternately to flex and extend the limb at the elbow.

4.2 The Foreleg

Holding the paw in one hand, massage the long flexor and extensor muscles of the foreleg for about a minute, making circular, kneading movements with the limb between your fingers and thumb. Grasp the limb in your right hand and give deep kneading massage (petrissage) in a rhythmic, circular pattern.

Work up from the carpus to the elbow. Finally, pull and push the leg alternately to flex and extend the limb at the elbow, after having first given several deep strokes and squeezes around the elbow joint where several muscles are attached. This will help loosen the elbow joint, which especially in older and heavy animals, can become a point of chronic lameness.

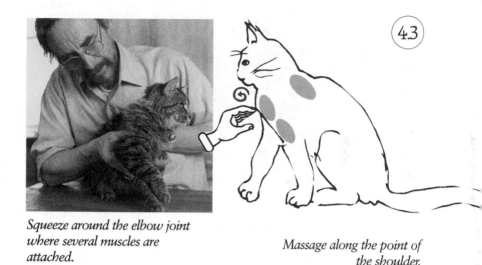

Squeeze around the elbow joint where several muscles are attached.

Massage along the point of the shoulder.

4.3 The Shoulder

With the foreleg (radius-ulna region) held firmly in one hand, massage the triceps, biceps, and other muscles that lie over the humerus for about one minute, again using fingers and thumb to create a rhythmic, circular, kneading massage pattern (petrissage). (See chart, page 49.)

Move up from the elbow to the point of the shoulder, flexing and extending the leg to help you locate the point of the shoulder. Pay particular attention to massaging across the point of the shoulder. As with each limb joint, it is advisable to make repeated slow, deep strokes across the joint over the tendons and muscles, which will help relax and tonify the muscles at these critical points of attachment. If the shoulder region is stiff, apply effleurage first, followed by fingertip massage before giving deeper petrissage.

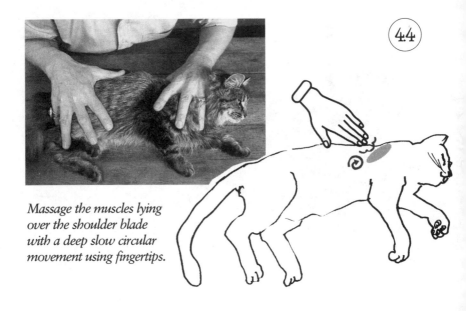

Massage the muscles lying over the shoulder blade with a deep slow circular movement using fingertips.

4.4 The Shoulder Blade (Scapula)

With the animal on its side, as usual, massage again for about one minute the muscles lying over the shoulder blade (scapula), with a deep, slow circular movement using fingertips. Locate the scapula by feeling for its upper edge and the ridge that runs down the center of it with the scapular muscles lying on each side.

Finally, apply acupressure to the ki points of the shoulder and forelimb and finish with a few superficial (effleurage) strokes. Turn the animal over and do the same to the other foreleg.

STEP FIVE: CHEST AND ABDOMEN

5.1 The Chest

Place the animal, sitting or lying, on one side. Give fingertip massage first on one side of the chest and then on the other. Keep your

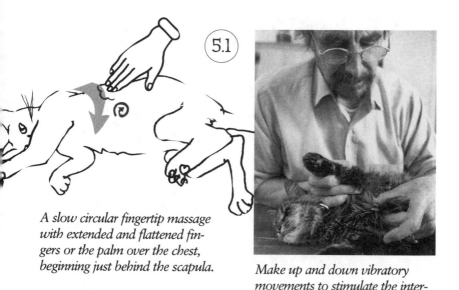

A slow circular fingertip massage
with extended and flattened fingers or the palm over the chest,
beginning just behind the scapula.

Make up and down vibratory
movements to stimulate the intercostal muscles between the ribs.

left hand on the animal's head, shoulder, or hip to keep it quiet and
relaxed at all times.

Then, begin a slow, circular fingertip massage for about one
minute with extended and flattened fingers or the palm of each
hand, over the chest, beginning just behind the scapula. You will be
massaging the fan-shaped latissimus muscle. Continue this same
pattern of light kneading or fingertip massage over your pet's entire
chest area. If the animal is sitting up, you may massage both sides
of the thorax with one hand on each side.

Massage between the ribs with one finger, making up and down
vibratory movements to stimulate the intercostal muscles between
the ribs. Follow each rib down from the spinal column to its
attachment at the sternum, or breastbone. Finally, give several light
strokes across the ribs, following the line of the fur.

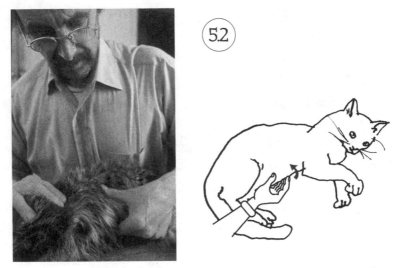

Hold the abdomen between flattened and extended fingers on one side and the thumb on the other.

5.2 The Abdomen

You can massage the abdomen with both hands, but for smaller animals you might want to hold the abdomen between flattened and extended fingers on one side and the thumb on the other.

Make slow, very gentle kneading movements, softly squeezing and relaxing the pressure between thumb and fingers, but never poking with thumb or fingers or pressing too hard. Continue for one minute.

Pressure near the pelvis may cause some discomfort if the cat has a full bladder or bladder infection. A lump may be felt near the lumbar vertebrae. This will most probably be one of the animal's kidneys and is no point for alarm. Pain in this region could mean kidney disease. (See Chapter 7.)

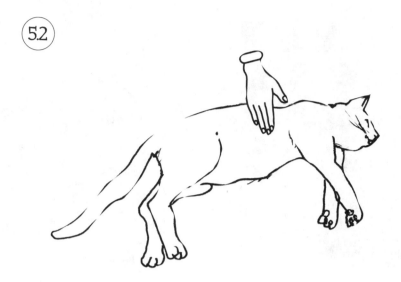

(5.2)

STEP SIX: HIP AND HIND LEG

Follow the same massage routine as with the foreleg for about the same duration, first kneading the foot while holding the leg with the other hand. Then, with one hand holding the foot, work up the leg slowly with the other hand. Note the anatomical differences between front and hind legs. Pay special attention to massaging around the tarsus or hock and along the Achilles tendon and especially where it attaches to the hock. Also, massage with fingers and thumb around the ligaments of the knee joint and patella or kneecap.

1. The Thigh

The muscles of the thigh, such as the biceps femoris and the gracilis, can take considerable deep massage. (See chart, page 49.)

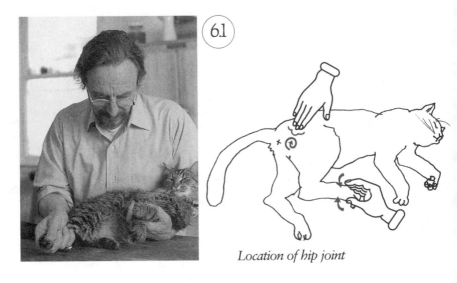

Location of hip joint

Knead the foot while holding the leg with the other hand. Flex and extend leg occasionally while working on the thigh muscles.

Flex and extend the leg occasionally while working on these muscles. You should be able to feel, inside the thigh when you press against the femur with your fingers, a clear, strong pulse. This is the femoral artery, which is most often used to take an animal's pulse.

Locate the hip joint by flexing and extending the hind leg and massage in a circular pattern around the hip region with fingertips. Follow this with acupressure to the ki points of the hind limb; give a few light strokes (effleurage) and then turn the animal over and massage the other hind leg.

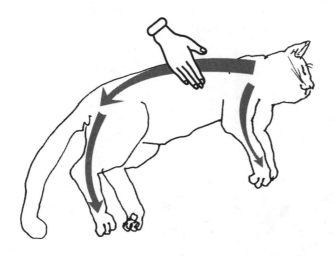

Finishing the massage

CLOSURE

Finish the regular massage treatment with slow palm and finger strokes from the head down the back to the sacrum, and from hip to hind foot and shoulder to forepaw, talking to your pet in a gentle and affectionate tone for about thirty seconds. There is no need to turn the animal over to repeat these closing strokes on the other side.

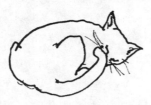

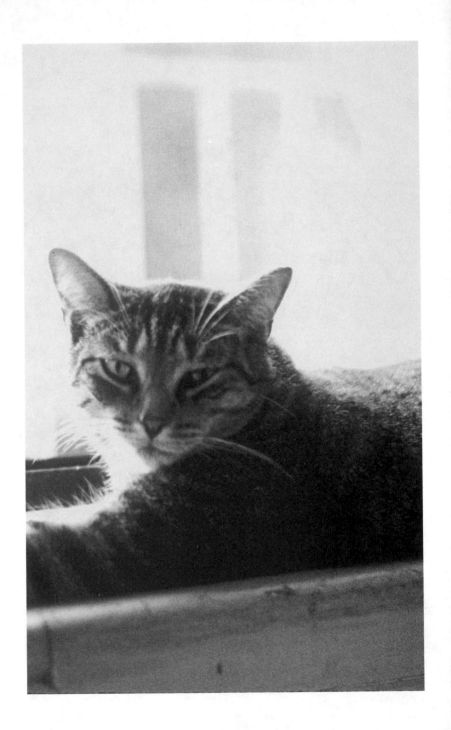

DIAGNOSTIC MASSAGE

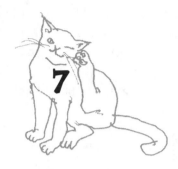

It is a fact of veterinary practice that too many owners bring their pets in for treatment days, even weeks, after the onset of an ailment. This used to make me furious, leaving me with the impression that many pet owners were uncaring and indifferent. However, with more experience, I saw how concerned these owners really were and how guilty they felt when I pointed out the passing of time had made the problem more serious, and I changed my views completely.

Pet owners are not uncaring and indifferent—quite the opposite, in fact. The problem, I discovered, was that few of them made a habit of carefully checking out their cat every week. And I don't mean giving them once-a-week or everyday grooming with a brush—that won't suffice. You have to feel and "see" with your hands. Your fingers have to search. And what method of checkup would be better than a diagnostic massage, which soothes and searches at once?

Of course, it is also possible and probable that you will pick up a problem during general massage when pressure or some manipulation causes your pet some discomfort. While regular massage can be of diagnostic help, what is really needed, and what you should give your pet at least once a week, is a thorough, rapid diagnostic massage.

A diagnostic massage goes much faster than regular massage. You can skip most of the deep manipulations described in the regular massage routine for cats, simply feeling the animal over for any abnormality. As you become more experienced, the diagnostic massage will become faster and faster and your touch lighter and more sensitive.

What are you looking for? Signs of pain, heat, swelling, or atrophy (shrinkage). If you are not sure that the suspect area is abnormally swollen or atrophied, compare it with the complementary opposite side of the animal. Remember, giving your pet a diagnostic massage will accustom it to examination, making it much easier for the veterinarian to examine your animal and treat it.

DIAGNOSTIC MASSAGE

Using the same palpating and exploring finger movements of circular massage and of petrissage described in the preceding chapter, follow the routine sequence (see page 56) as given for the general massage, so you won't miss any part of the body.

Whenever you locate a diagnostic point that leads you to suspect any abnormality, consult your veterinarian for further advice: do not try to home-doctor without veterinary supervision, and give no further massage until you get your vet's okay.

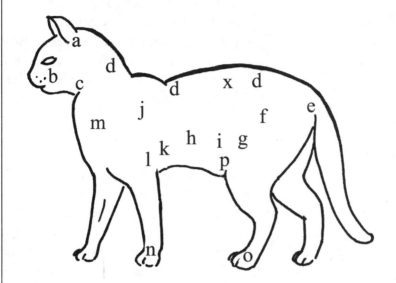

Some of the diagnostic pain points in the cat

Pressure on these points elicits a pain response:

(a) ear–otitis or ear canal infection

(b) tooth abscess or gum infection

(c) pharyngitis or tonsillitis

(d) along back–intervertebral disk luxation, arthritis

(e) anal gland infection or impaction

(f) hip arthritis or dysplasia

(g) cystitis or bladder infection or obstruction

(h) abdominal pain–foreign body obstruction, infection, peritonitis

(i) low abdominal pain–hepatitis, pancreatitis

(j) chest region—pleurisy, pneumonia

(k) heart region—pericarditis, endocarditis

(l) elbow—arthritis, bursitis

(m) shoulder—arthritis

(n) forepaw—foreign body, cyst, or referred pain from l, m, k, or d

(o) hindpaw—foreign body, cyst, or referred pain from p, f, g, or d

(p) knee—patella dislocation or torn cruciate ligament

(x) kidney region—nephritis

HEAD AND NECK

Pay particular attention to how your cat reacts to pressure at any of the diagnostic and pain points that will be shortly described.

Check also if there is any discharge from the nose, eyes, or ears, which could indicate a local infection or inflammation. In cats, discharge of this kind could signify a serious vital disease needing veterinary treatment. Clean the discharge with water-moistened cotton.

1. The Ear

The base of the ear is a diagnostic key point. If the animal feels pain there when pressed with thumb or forefinger, that could signify an ear infection. Violent head shaking or scratching of the ear with one hind leg can occur in the absence of any ear problem, but can also indicate your cat has ear mites or an ear infection and requires a visit to the vet. A tarry, brown discharge is a sure sign of ear mites. Probe into the ear canal gently with a cotton-tipped swab. It should not come out smelling unpleasant or with anything more than a little clear cerumen (ear wax) on it.

Feel both ear flaps. Heat and swelling could mean your cat is developing a blood blister, or hematoma; it will eventually be resorbed and make the ear shrivel up and look deformed. Such hematomas are often associated with ear mites or ear canal infection, caused by your pet scratching its ear and shaking its head violently. Blood blisters require veterinary treatment to stop them from enlarging.

2. The Neck

Pain or pressure at the back of the neck can mean that your pet has a vertebral disk or other spinal disorder, especially if it seems to have pain walking or favors one foreleg. Point this out to your vet on your next visit. If the animal exhibits signs of great pain, see the vet immediately.

Always palpate gently with your fingers around the animal's throat and behind the angle of each jaw. Try to locate the neck lymph glands. (See charts, page 90.) In cats, these are located in approximately the same place as ours, and, as with us, these glands swell when the animal has a sore throat or other disorders. Any marked swelling on either or both sides or a sudden increase in size of these glands, warrants a visit to the veterinarian. Swelling in this region could mean your pet has lymphatic cancer.

3. The Mouth

Open your cat's mouth and check the gums for signs of swelling and redness and the teeth for brown scale and tartar. Either or both of these cause gum infection and tooth loss and should be seen by the veterinarian. Brush your pet's teeth and massage its gums with your fingers if it has chronic dental problems.

Pain on pressing the side of the face around the roots of the upper teeth can be a sign of sinusitis in cats, or of an abscessed tooth.

THE THORAX, ABDOMEN, AND BACK
1. The Thorax

Pain when massaging or palpating the thorax (chest) can be a sign of a respiratory disorder such as pleurisy or pneumonia. It can also mean that the animal has received a blow on one side. Bruising is difficult to detect in an animal, but slight swelling and tenderness are cardinal signs.

2. The Abdomen

An animal that has difficulty breathing could be suffering from a number of problems, including heart disease or respiratory infection. If the abdomen is also swollen and the animal has poor exercise tolerance, it most likely is suffering from congestive heart failure. Gentle, regular massage plus digitalis medication will help many geriatric pets with this disorder. A special diet and frequent veterinary checkups are also indicated.

The swollen abdomen in heart failure is due to the build-up of ascitic fluid. This can be felt as a soggy mass when the abdomen is palpated, and it can be felt with the palm of one hand on one flank when the other side is tapped sharply with a finger. Abdominal swelling can also mean pregnancy; after five or six weeks the developing fetuses should be easily felt, and in lean animals their movements are visible when the mother is lying on one side.

Abdominal swelling and pain can mean infectious peritonitis, a prevalent disease in cats. A small swelling in the midline—the middle of the abdomen—could be either the scar of the umbilicus, or navel, or an umbilical hernia. In some pets, a large hernia may be felt under the fur. This should generally be corrected, since the bowels could get caught in it and serious complications ensue.

Other hernias can be felt in the cat's inguinal or groin region. A large mass of soft tissue in the groin that seems to disappear when it is gently pushed in is most likely intestines that have herniated. Corrective surgery is advisable. A somewhat similar mass can be felt in cats in each groin, but this is only subcutaneous and deep fat, and it is quite natural for mature cats to develop such fat folds in the groin region.

When giving a diagnostic massage to an animal, I like to lift up the hind legs and check the hips for symmetry. If one leg is shorter than the other, or one side of the rump or thigh thinner, then arthritis, prior injury, or hip dysplasia is suspect. Report this to your animal doctor. If the animal has difficulty in breathing when held in this position, it should see the veterinarian at once, since it could have a diaphragmatic hernia.

The abdomen should feel soft and resilient when gently palpated, and if the animal suddenly tenses its abdominal muscles, this can mean that you are handling it too roughly, that it is afraid, or that it has some problem in the abdomen, such as a painfully enlarged liver, a bowel obstruction, or even a tumor. If in doubt, don't poke around because you could cause further complications. See your veterinarian. Rough and inexperienced handling of the abdomen could cause a blocked bladder to burst, and then the animal has little hope. Tenderness in the lower or posterior abdominal area near the rim of the pelvis could mean that your animal has a bladder or uterine infection.

Always visually inspect the animal's external genitals and palpate the testicles. The genitals should appear pink and moist without any discolored discharge. Danger signals to report to the vet: a brownish discharge from a female cat (it may indicate uterine infection or pyometra); one testicle being larger than the other (it could mean that a tumor is developing).

Always carefully examine the nipples and mammary (breast) tissue when giving a diagnostic or general massage to a female cat. Squeeze each nipple and note any discolored brownish or greenish discharge that could mean infection. Swelling of the gland tissue could mean pregnancy or false pregnancy; it could also signal that breast tumors are developing. Hard lumps will develop in the breast tissue as the tumors become more obvious. Surgical treatment is advisable to stop the spread of the cancer to internal organs. Routine diagnostic massage could turn up earlier detection of mammary tumors or cancer, and give your cat a better chance of recovery.

3. The Back

Tenderness at any of the ki or association points (see chart, page 105) along the back can be indicative of a vertebral disk problem or internal disorder, such as kidney disease or nephritis. Pain in the back region from some internal disorder is termed referred pain. A classic example in man is angina pectoris, pain in the armpit and arm referred from heart disease.

Pain, when massaging around the base of the tail or rump region, could be referred from impacted or infected anal glands, a common affliction in cats. Pain, while the animal is defecating and while it is being palpated in the pelvic region, could be a sign of constipation, or tumor. A swelling on one side of the anus sometimes develops and this is a hernia, often caused by the animal straining because an enlarged prostate is making it difficult to defecate. All these conditions need veterinary consultation.

Always check your cat's tail, running the hand down it and feeling each coccygeal or tail vertebra. Pain and/or swelling can mean either a crush wound, from being trapped in a door, for instance, or a bite wound. These wounds should be treated to avoid complications.

4. The Skin

After routine diagnostic massage of the thorax, abdomen, and back, ruffle the animal's hair and roll the skin all over between your fingers and thumbs to check it for tumors, external parasites, signs of eczema, alopecia (baldness), or other dermatological problems.

When the skin does not feel elastic but tends to stay in position where it has been squeezed, then the animal is most likely sick, suffering from dehydration, and needs a doctor.

Areas of skin that feel cool and are losing fur may be symptomatic of thyroid insufficiency or other hormonal disorder. Report your findings to the vet; medication can control these conditions.

To finish off, using the palms of the hands and extended fingers, smooth the fur back in place with brisk strokes from head to rump.

FORELEGS AND HIND LEGS

Again, search or "feel-see" with your fingers as you quickly palpate and knead each leg, beginning with the paw and working systematically up the limb, then to the scapula or hip region.

Be alert for painful hot swellings, particularly along the radius and ulna. These will most likely be bite abscesses and may need veterinary treatment, especially if the cat is off its food and has a fever.

WARNING POINTS
To "Feel-See" with Your Fingers

• *Swelling* under the skin. This could mean bite abscesses—or one of many forms of cancer.

• *Pain* upon pressure near the ears or on the face. This could signal a chronic ear infection or an abscessed tooth.

• *Tenderness* along the back. This could indicate kidney disease or a slipped disc. Heat, as in a paw or ear, could mean infection.

• *Cold*, as in a paw, could mean blocked circulation.

• Feeling for *moistness, dryness, suppleness,* and *oiliness* in the animal's coat is also of diagnostic value.

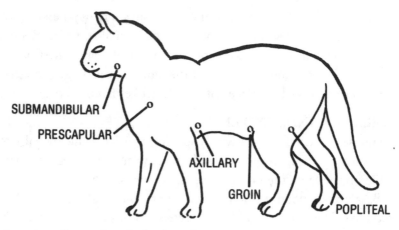

Location of major lymph glands in the cat

Note any pain or swelling around the joints, or distress when the limb is extended or flexed. These could be signs of arthritis, hip or elbow dysplasia, or a torn cruciate (knee) ligament. The degree of distress will determine if it's an emergency or can be reported at your next veterinary visit.

Painless swelling (edema) of the limbs is a sign of cardiac malfunction, and, as in humans, benefits from massage and from a diet low in sodium salt. Edematous swelling will pit on pressure; the indentation will remain for several seconds after the finger is removed. If you detect such swelling, check the mucous membranes of the mouth. They may be bluish rather than pink, an indication of inadequate circulation and oxygenation, called cyanosis. Get advice from your veterinarian, of course. (In jaundice conditions associated with liver disorders, these membranes have a yellowish tinge, and in shock or anemia they are pale and the capillaries in the lips do not fill up quickly or turn pink after being pressed between the fingers.)

Look out for any signs of hard swelling on the long bones, especially near the epiphyses or ends of the bones.

Heat and pain between the toes could be a sign of interdigital cysts, especially if the cat has been licking or chewing its foot or feet.

THE GLANDS
Familiarize yourself with the location of the major lymph glands and always "feel-see" these when giving your pet its weekly diagnostic massage.

Check the glands in the maxillary, or throat, area, the axilla, or armpit, groin, prescapular, and upper hock areas. General enlargement can mean lymphatic cancer; local enlargement of maxillary or prescapular lymph glands could be a sign of infection in that area, such as an infected tooth or bite wound on the front paw.

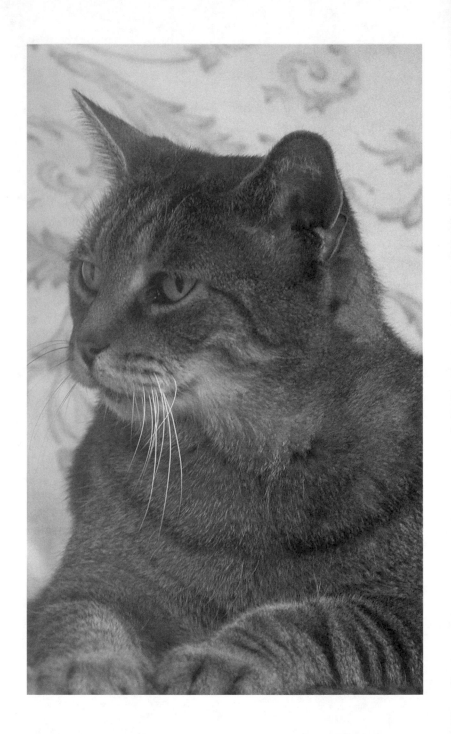

THERAPEUTIC MASSAGE

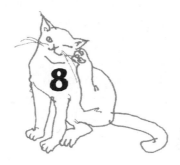

Since general massage is regarded as an ingredient of health care maintenance or preventive medicine, when used appropriately it is therapeutic massage, per se. Therefore, with a sick pet, you apply the general massage sequence delineated in Chapter 6, keeping in mind certain precautions which I will point out to you, and also adding certain procedures for specific conditions.

The therapeutic massage that I have developed consists of three parts. First, the general massage as outlined in Chapter 6. Secondly, a massage pattern specific for the particular condition you wish to alleviate. And thirdly, the laying on of "healing hands," which, in the opinion of some human massage therapists and psychic healers, is the most beneficial procedure of all. No massage therapy should be given, however, if it does not meet with your animal doctor's approval or if, as will be described, the animal's condition could be aggravated by massage manipulations.

The strokes and fingertip manipulations you use will vary according to your pet's particular problem. They include the entire spectrum of manipulations, such as thumb and fingertip acupressure, effleurage and petrissage, circular fingertip massage, and friction massage, as described in Chapter 6.

In the laying on of hands, you simply place your hands around or above and below the injured or diseased part. As you breathe in, imagine that you are drawing out the pain, inflammation, or sickness, and as you breathe out, envision the life force or healing energy (ki) flowing out through your hands and into the animal. Laying on of hands can be done after a general or local therapeutic massage and also on pets whose condition rules out giving any form of therapeutic massage, such as extremely sick comatose animals and those suffering from fever, shock, severe trauma, infection, or poisoning.

Also, visualize the afflicted part or body system returning to its normal state. Visualization is a self-help healing technique that is attracting a lot of medical interest. It may also be used by the healer.

General therapeutic massage outlined in this chapter will help in the following cases:

- recovery from sickness

- recovery from surgery

- circulatory disorders, especially
  impaired heart functions in old age

- hypothyroidism

- obesity

- impaired liver function

- impaired kidney function

- musculo-skeletal problems such as sprains, and hip dysplasia

There are some conditions that should not receive any local massage in the vicinity of the ailment. The only therapeutic contact should be the laying on of hands and light effleurage and fingertip massage. These conditions (which should be receiving veterinary attention) include:

- recent fractures

- ruptured vertebral disks

- recent sprains and torn muscles and ligaments

- acute inflammations, as from a bite or skin infection (massage might spread the infection)

- swellings, such as blood blisters (hematomas)

- enlarged lymph glands

- cuts, bruises, or recent abrasions or fresh scar tissue

- any area that seems unusually tender (and if you can't figure out what the problem is, take your pet to the veterinarian)

Never massage an animal that has a fever, is in a state of shock, extreme debility, or has heat stroke. Consult your veterinarian or local veterinary emergency service without delay.

After surgery, avoid massaging near or over the incision area.

Place sick or debilitated pets on a soft blanket or foam-rubber pad. If the room is cold, an electric heater pad may be comforting and relaxing to muscles.

Be sure that you position yourself so that you don't have to reach out or bend too much to massage your pet. It is important for you to be as comfortable as your animal patient.

GENERAL THERAPEUTIC MASSAGE

Follow the same sequence and timing as outlined in Chapter 6, paying particular attention to the following manipulations:

Start with the back region and then follow the same sequence as described in Chapter 6. Give effleurage, then fingertip massage, then petrissage, and finally acupressure for each region, and finish with closure strokes and a laying on of hands.

1. Effleurage

Begin therapeutic massage with effleurage—a light stroking technique (see Chapter 6). The animal will get used to your touch, and at the same time you can explore for signs of soreness or swelling, as outlined in Chapter 7, which deals with diagnostic massage. Keep the strokes light and slow at first to calm or sedate the animal, and then increase the pressure.

Effleurage should be given to sick animals from the periphery to the center and is centripetal, moving up from the hips to the chest, and from hind foot to hip to invigorate, and in the opposite direction to calm. The rhythm of lighter strokes can be anywhere from fifteen to thirty per minute and for slower, deeper ones, as low as five to ten per minute. Continue this massage for about five minutes.

For tense, anxious animals, use a slow gentle rhythm, adjusting the pressure of each stroke so that it does not cause pain. The direction of massage on the legs should be away from the body, beginning at the hip or shoulder and working down to the feet. A slow rhythmic massage is relaxing, while a more vigorous rhythm is stimulating.

For convalescing pets and aged pets suffering from chronic debilitating diseases, give a stimulating tonifying massage, using proportionately more fingertip circular massage strokes and less effleurage in order to increase the rate of venous return of the blood circulation. The rhythm is faster, and the pressure is deeper and shorter.

2. Petrissage or Deep Massage

Follow effleurage and fingertip massage with petrissage. Petrissage is a combination of kneading, twisting, pulling, and rolling movements made with your fingers and thumbs and palms of your hands. (See Chapter 6.) Instead of gently and slowly sliding as in the more superficial effleurage, petrissage picks up and then rolls, wrings, and compresses skin and muscles. This stimulates both the muscular and lymphatic systems and helps loosen scar tissue, contracted muscles, and tight tendons. Five to ten minutes is sufficient.

The patient must be relaxed for this deep massage for, if tense, petrissage is difficult. If petrissage is too hard or painful, a protective muscle contraction will be felt. Ease off at once and proceed more gently.

Deep massage into the connective tissue and fat can do two things. As in Rolfing—a deep-pressure massage system developed by Ida P. Rolf—it can result in the release of toxins stored in the fat (and the smell on a patient's breath and skin can be terrible).

Deep massage will help stimulate the circulation of blood in the veins and lymph in the lymphatic system.

3. Acupressure

The next step in general therapeutic massage is acupressure (described in Chapters 6 and 7). Be careful to avoid acupressure around painful or inflamed areas until you and your pet are confident and you can "feel-see" with your fingers. Then try very gently to apply direct through-and-through pressure to the acupressure point.

Do not press hard with finger or thumb. Begin by feeling for the round, softly palpable but seemingly imaginary acupressure points. Make searching, circular movements and the point will find you. Then make circular movements clockwise, gradually increasing the pressure and holding it for about thirty seconds as you breathe out and send your ki into the ki point of your patient. This will help tonify and increase the rate of healing. Reversing the movement is said to help reduce inflammations by drawing excess ki away, and you should make this reverse movement as you are breathing in, according to some human acupressure therapists. Personally, I find little difference, provided the ki points receive some external stimulation.

Once you feel you have mastered this acupressure technique, you can build it into your therapeutic routine as follows: give five minutes' relaxation and effleurage, followed by five minutes' general petrissage and then five minutes of acupressure. Then give five minutes' attention to a specific problem area as I will now describe. And then finish with a five-minute closure period.

4. Localized Therapeutic Massage

For cats with some localized ailment, such as an arthritic hip or sprained leg, give the general body massage as described in Chapter 6, followed by localized therapeutic massage.

Proceed to the specific area of concern, such as a sore knee or arthritic hip for three to four minutes of concentrated, localized massage. (Descriptions follow in next section.)

5. Fingertip Massage

After this, I like to give a quick fingertip massage all over for about one minute. This is the rhythmic massage using fingertips and moderate pressure, making small circular movements. The fingers stay on the skin all the time, making four or five quick, small circles before moving to an adjacent spot.

6. Completion of Sequence

Terminate the therapeutic massage sequence with a very light effleurage, simply passing the hands gently over the body and limbs, and then give a laying on of the hands if you wish, visualizing a whole and healthy body that your skill and love helped to restore.

SPECIFIC (LOCALIZED) THERAPEUTIC MASSAGE

Specific localized massage is very helpful for sprains, torn ligaments and muscles, arthritis, localized trauma from an automobile or other injury, once the primary healing processes have begun.

Localized therapeutic massage for five to ten minutes once or twice daily helps break down fibrous tissue adhesions. It also increases the rate of exchange of arterial and venous blood and of lymph circulation, thus speeding up the removal of waste products and accelerating the rate of healing. Use a combination of fingertip circular massage and deeper petrissage, remembering to go lightly where there is pain and working across the lie of the tendons and muscles for maximal effect.

Sprains, chronic arthritis, or *old joint injury*: Massage is not a cure, but it will take away some of the cat's pain and stiffness, especially if it is done early in the day.

A cat suffering from any of a number of chronic diseases involving the back, hips, or shoulders will benefit greatly from a daily therapeutic massage. Follow the sequential procedure outlined above, namely five minutes' relaxing effleurage and five minutes' firm petrissage all over the body. Then follow this with five minutes' deep petrissage and acupressure around the neck, shoulders, thighs, hips, and lower back respectively. Pay particular attention to any afflicted joint area and to weak atrophying muscles and fibrous knots or adhesions. Intersperse this treatment by flexing and extending the leg to help tonify and reflexively relax the leg musculature. Then give the closure sequence of general body friction rub and light passing over of hands. If you are not sure what the afflicted area should feel like, check the other, presumably normal side of the animal, as a reference point for comparison if the problem affects only one side of the body. Always press the skin and tissues beneath lightly when you feel bony prominences, because such points can be quite sensitive. Friction massage is also effective in such areas.

Similar treatment can be given for local strains, sprains, and torn ligaments, especially of the knee, or patella, region, once the swelling and initial pain have subsided.

Massage can be safer than giving drugs such as cortisone for prolonged periods. These can have serious side effects, resulting in so-called iatrogenic diseases. When properly done, massage has no such negative consequences, and can also be used as an adjunct to appropriate drug and other treatments.

Animals, like human patients undergoing massage, may sometimes experience transient dizziness or sleepiness and occasionally nausea. These relate, I believe, to the freeing of toxins in the tissues as a result of direct physical manipulation and enhanced local circulation. They may also be due to the release of endorphins and other "feel-good" substances from the body.

It is also at the ends of the bones that growth is taking place (at the so-called growth plates or epiphyses of the longbones just behind the knob ends that form the joints). Massage here will help the circulation, which in turn will aid in the proper calcification and growth of the limbs.

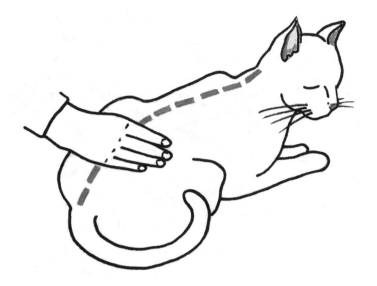

Deep petrissage and acupressure around the neck, shoulders, thighs, hips, and lower back

---

Each limb should also be extended and flexed repeatedly (10–20 times) to move the joints and tendons and reflexively relax antagonistic muscles.

For impaired heart function in old age (with or without peripheral edema or swelling), pay particular attention to massaging the extremities with effleurage, beginning at the toes and working up to stimulate the circulation and help the lymphatic circulation.

Give the animal five minutes of general relaxing effleurage, then five minutes' gentle, "soft" rather than firm petrissage, followed by five minutes of tonifying acupressure; then close with sixty seconds of invigorating friction massage all over the body and light effleurage.

Generally, I am opposed to the use of electrical vibrators for therapeutic massage, preferring the direct hands-on and laying-on-of-hands approach. However, many physical disorders, such as arthritis of both people and pets, respond well to other physio-therapy techniques, such as deep-heat treatment (microwave and short-wave diathermy) and ultrasound.

ACUPUNCTURE AND ACUPRESSURE THERAPY

Acupuncture is also effective on pets for a number of disorders, and there is now the American Association of Veterinary Acupuncturists, all graduate veterinarians who are exploring some of the "new frontiers" of Western medicine, many of which, like acupuncture, are very ancient techniques that predate most, if not all, contemporary Western medicine's techniques and philosophy.

There are several ki points called master points, source points, and alarm points that are stimulated and read for diagnosis in acupuncture therapy. Giving some acupressure massage to these points may provide additional benefit when giving a routine, as well as a therapeutic, massage. These points, however, take considerable experience and skill to locate and are best left to trained veterinary acupuncture specialists. A routine massage, following the sequence outlined below and providing the right kind of pressure through appropriate strokes over the body surface, will stimulate many of these ki points anyway. This is probably an additional reason for the beneficial and therapeutic effects of the routine massage that I have given in this book.

There are some forty major acupuncture points identified in animals that can be stimulated to help alleviate a number of conditions, ranging from increasing production of antibodies and body resistance to disease, to treating eczema, arthritis, respiratory diseases, shock, and also digestive, circulatory, and renal disorders.

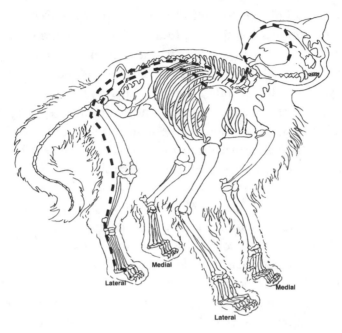

Lateral

Medial

Medial

Lateral

The Bladder Meridian

Acupuncture is used mainly to relieve pain and, too, for its effects on the autonomic nervous system. Further veterinary research is making acupuncture diagnosis and therapy more widely accepted by the profession and more readily available for sick or injured pets. Since massage can help stimulate some of these ki points and also has beneficial effects on the physiological system in times of sickness, therapeutic massage is one way for the pet owner to assist the veterinarian in restoring a pet's health when it is sick or injured and keeping the animal healthy, as part of a total health-care program.

GUIDE TO FELINE ACUPRESSURE MAINTENANCE

Start by finding a comfortable location for you and your cat. The location needs to be a place where it is calm and you can relax. Slowly, take five breaths in and out. Think about how you want to help your cat feel healthy and energetically balanced. Taking a moment to formulate the intent of your treatment is very important.

Begin by resting one hand on the animal's shoulder. Using the heel of your other hand, place it at the top of your animal's head and gently (one to two pounds of pressure) stroke down his neck, just off the midline. For very small animals, use your index and second fingers to trace from the top of his head down his neck, staying just off the animal's midline. Follow the diagram for the Bladder Meridian on the previous page. Continue stroking down to the hindquarters, staying to the side of the midline.

To finish, stroke down along the outside of your cat's leg to the tip of his outside toe. Your opposite hand can trail along the same path gliding gently. Repeat this intentional stroking procedure three times on each side following the Bladder Meridian located on both sides of the spine.

Now you are ready for Point Work. Rest one hand on your cat wherever it feels comfortable. This is your anchor hand and you can move it whenever you need to for comfort. (It is good to have both hands on the animal throughout the Point Work segment of the treatment for two reasons: You will be able to feel the cat's reactions to the Point Work and it is more settling for the animal.) You will be performing the actual point work with your other hand.

The acupressure points identified in the chart on the next page help balance Chi (also known as Ki, pronounced "chee"), the life-force energy throughout the cat's body, and they boost the immune system. The harmonious and free flow of Chi in the body supports the animal's immune system and keeps his body healthy and strong.

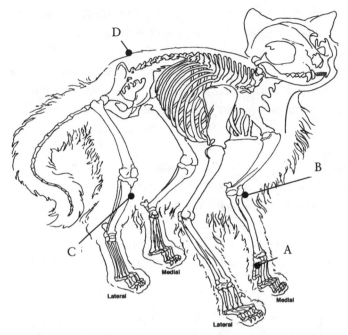

Feline Health Maintenance Acupressure Treatment—Point Work

A. This point is located at the webbing of the dew-claw on the
   forearm.

B. This acupoint is located in the crease of the elbow. Lift the
   cat's forearm, then run your finger along the lateral crease
   at the elbow joint and you will feel a little indentation.

C. Located on the front and lateral side of the hind leg, about
   1/2 to 1 inch below the stifle (knee).

D. Located on the dorsal midline at the lumbosacral space.
   This is a good acupoint to stimulate by light scratching at
   the end of the treatment.

You can use either the thumb or two-finger technique to perform Point Work, depending on what is most comfortable for you.

• **Thumb technique.** Place the fleshy tip of your thumb directly on the acupressure point at a 90-degree angle, also called "acupoint," and hold the point gently, but with intent, for three to five deep breaths. Try to pattern your breathing with your cat.

• **Two-finger technique.** Put your middle finger on top of your index finger, and then place your index finger at approximately a 90-degree angle gently, but with intentional firmness, and directly on the acupressure point for three to five breaths. Try to pattern your breathing with the animal. The two-finger technique tends to work best for smaller animals and in places that are difficult to reach.

Since the body is bilateral, once you have finished holding the acupressure points on one side of your cat, be sure to hold the points on the other side. Doing both sides will ensure a balanced and more complete treatment.

Watch your pet's reaction to the Point Work. Healthy energy releases are: yawning, deep breathing, muscle twitches, release of air, deeper relaxation, licking, and softening of the eye. If your cat is overly reactive to a particular point or exhibits a pain reaction, work in front of or behind the acupressure point that was reactive. Try that point again at a later session if it bothers your animal too much and detracts from the treatment.

To complete your treatment session, rest your hand comfortably on your pet's shoulder just the way you did when starting the treatment. Place the heel of your other hand, or index and middle fingers, just off the midline of the top of his head and stroke down his neck, over his back to his hindquarters, keeping your hand to the side of his spine, and down the outside of his leg to his outer toe. You are tracing the Bladder Meridian. Your opposite hand can lightly trail along the same path as the working hand. Repeat this procedure three times on each side of your cat. It can take 24 hours for the effects of an acupressure treatment to be fully experienced.

[Contributed by Nancy Zidonis and Amy Snow, authors of *The Well-Connected Dog: A Guide to Canine Acupressure*; *Acu-Cat: A Guide to Feline Acupressure*; and *Equine Acupressure: A Working Manual*. They own Tallgrass Publishers, which offers Meridian charts for dogs, cats, and horses, plus *Introducing Equine Acupressure*, a 50-minute training video. Tallgrass Animal Acupressure provides training courses worldwide.

To contact them, phone: 888-841-7211, or on the web: www.animalacupressure.com; email: acupressure4all@earthlink.net]

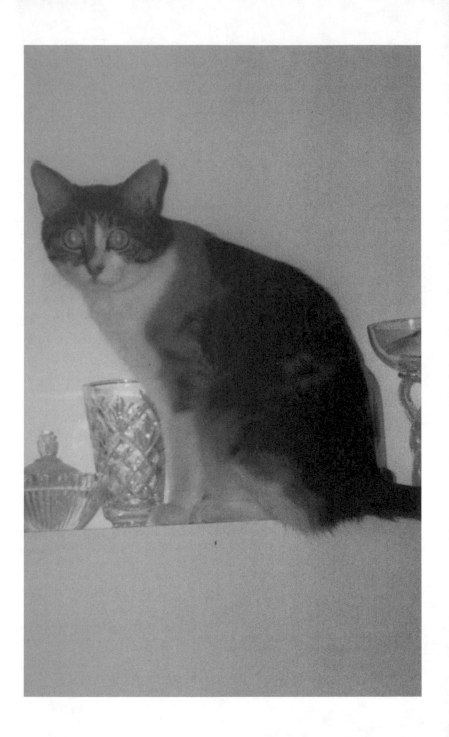

TOTAL HEALTH CARE
FOR CATS

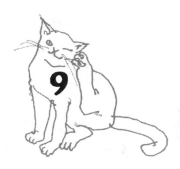

Your cat has certain inalienable rights: foremost among them is the right to health care. To achieve and maintain total health for your cat, you should follow a program of preventive medicine.

Preventive medicine is the best medicine. In both human and veterinary medicine today we need to banish the notion that health is the absence of disease. A more positive view is needed, otherwise symptoms alone will be treated and not the causes. Health is not the absence of disease: It is well-being, both physical and psychological. Our lifestyles, habits, attitudes, temperament, and relationships with others (especially in the family) influence our overall well-being and health. The same is true for our pets. Similarly, what we feed our pets and how we take care of their basic health requirements have a significant influence on the animal's health and resistance to stress and disease.

The following key elements make up a holistic health ritual to keep your cat in top shape. Use it as a constant reminder. Whenever possible, I have written it in the form of a checklist for easy reference.

REGULAR CHECKUPS

- New kittens need a thorough going-over by the veterinarian.

- Adult cats should have a total checkup at least once a year.

- Cats are prone to virus infections, which often appear as a "cold" or a total loss of appetite.

- Cystitis, or urinary bladder disease, is also very prevalent, and can result in painful urination or a sudden blockage of the urethra, especially in male cats. Be alert to the following symptoms: straining to urinate, a distended bladder (which can easily be felt with diagnostic massage), and blood in the urine. Cystitis is a veterinary emergency.

SIGNS OF ILLNESS IN YOUR CAT
(requiring veterinary attention)

- Sits quietly in a hunched-up position and remains inactive

- Stops grooming itself

- Coat appears dull and seems to "stand up"

- Sore gums, bad breath

- Goes off its regular food

- Suffers diarrhea for more than 24 hours

- Shows difficulty urinating

- Shows difficulty breathing

- Vomits repeatedly

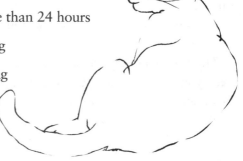

- Sneezes frequently, accompanied by a runny discharge from the eyes and/or nose

- Keeps scratching behind its ears, or shakes its head. Secretes a brown discharge in one or both ears. (This can signal ear mites, a common problem in cats.)

VACCINATIONS

- Kittens usually need a series of shots against the common virus diseases feline distemper (panleukopenia), pneumonitis, and cat "flu." Cats who never go outdoors need few, if any, vaccinations.

- New kittens (and other cats in the household) should be examined for the very serious cat diseases—feline viral leukemia, or cat distemper, and feline AIDS, a bite-transmitted immunodeficiency disease that is not communicable to humans.

- Adult cats need periodic "booster" shots; your vet will keep a record. Too many indoor cats who are never allowed to roam the neighborhood (nor should they, I believe) are given unnecessary vaccinations, because the risks far exceed the chances of exposure to infected cats.

- A rabies shot (three years duration) is advised for cats who go outdoors (at six months or later).

- Never vaccinate a sick, injured, pregnant, or nursing cat.

WORMING

- Take your kitten's stool sample to the vet to be checked out for roundworms. (Kittens are often born with this parasite.)

- Adult cats become infested with tapeworms from eating small rodents. Stools will show small, white rice-like particles. See your vet. Also be sure to fight fleas, since some tapeworms have part of their life cycle in the flea.

  CAUTION: Do not routinely worm your cat. If it becomes sick, consult your vet. Worming is no panacea, and can indeed be harmful if it leads you to ignore other symptoms.

FLEAS

- Ask your veterinarian to recommend a cat dip or powder for fleas. Never buy over-the-counter chemicals.

- Never use a flea medication that is prescribed for dogs; it may make your cat sick!

- Fleas spend part of their life cycle as grubs, living in floor crevices, carpets, etc. So vacuum your house thoroughly. If necessary, have the house fumigated by your local department of health. Use every natural method of flea control you can find, and put off as long as you can exposing your cat to any of these hazardous insecticidal poisons.

- Some cats are allergic to flea collars. Avoid using them at all costs.

- Keep your cat indoors; that way it won't get fleas, tapeworms, and/or other infectious diseases from neighboring cats. Cats who have never known the outdoors don't miss it much, compared to those who have, and are suddenly confined. Cats are quite happy on a leash outdoors for occasional fresh-air walks, and most enjoy being allowed outdoors into a cat-proof yard or enclosure.

MASSAGE

Your cat should receive a weekly massage (or more, if it seems to enjoy it!). Pay special attention to your cat's ears, teeth, gums, and upper respiratory system, since they are particularly susceptible to various infections, which will require veterinary attention.

GROOMING

- Cats do a good job of grooming themselves, but you must nonetheless brush long-haired cats daily, short-haired cats twice a week. Cats swallow fur and get fur balls as a result; brushing helps cut down on the amount of fur swallowed.

- If you see bald spots, check with your veterinarian. It may be a diet problem, an infection, an allergy, or an hormonal imbalance.

- Cats who roam out of the house may occasionally require a bath. Sponging with warm water and baby shampoo is the least traumatic for cats, who do not like to get wet. Rinse very well, because the residue may cause irritation. Towel-dry; keep the cat out of drafts while wet.

- House cats should have a scratching post, or they'll use their claws on your furniture, rugs, etc. Provide one early in life. Until your cat is trained to the post, trim its nails by holding the paw to the light and trimming down close to the "quick." Claw the post yourself with your nails to attract the cat and sprinkle catnip on the post.

- Remove wax from the cat's ears with a cloth-wrapped finger or a cotton swab dipped in oil. A foul odor means trouble.

- Cats are susceptible to gum disease; they don't get cavities but lose their teeth. Tartar (yellow-brown or gray-white hard deposits on the teeth) must be removed by a veterinarian. You can clean your cat's teeth regularly (once a week with a rough cloth). If the gums bleed, it is a sign of disease that needs treatment. Massaging the gums with circular motions (using your finger or a cotton swab) is helpful.

EXERCISE

- Play is the best form of exercise for cats. Games also make for "bonding" between the owner and his cat. Some suggested activities and games:

- A cat-mobile for the pet to swipe at.

- Hide-and-seek between owner and pet.

- A paper bag for the cat to explore.

- Tie a ball or lightweight toy on the end of a string; as the cat paws it, pull the string.

- Play retrieve-the-(small)-object, with Siamese cats especially.

- Best of all, have at least two cats. They really know how to play and communicate with each other and are generally brighter and healthier than felines in one-cat homes.

DIET FOR KITTENS

- Accomplish weaning gradually, ending anywhere from 10-12 weeks of age. Human-socialize gradually to avoid behavior problems later in life.

- Feed kittens (as well as cats) a complete and balanced, ideally organic or top quality commercial cat food; that way you are sure all nutritional demands are being met.

- Feedings:
  until 4 months . . . . 4 times a day

  4–6 months . . . . 3 times a day

  6 months on . . . . 2 times a day

- Feed *regularly* to achieve regular elimination and keep appetite wholesome.

- Stick to a core of basic recipes right from infancy on. That will keep your cat from becoming a finicky eater.

- Cow's milk may give your kitten diarrhea if he is intolerant of high levels of milk sugar (lactose); be alert!

- An all-meat or all-fish diet is unbalanced and can cause nutritional disorders in kittens.

ADULT CATS

- Feed your cat a scientifically analyzed and formulated reputable brand of canned or fresh-frozen commercial cat food, which provides necessary vitamins, minerals, and protein. Avoid several serious health problems such as obesity, cystitis, and diabetes by never feeding your cat exclusively on a diet of dry or semi-moist food.

- You may want to try feeding your cat some raw foods—meats, poultry, fish, fruits, and vegetables. Or make up balanced meals from home-prepared ingredients.

- Cats do enjoy table scraps of fish or chicken, but don't give more than one-quarter of its diet in such treats.

- Provide a little dry food for the cat to chew at will; it helps keep feline teeth clean. Chewing on raw chicken wings also helps.

- Don't hinder your cat from eating grass; it's an excellent internal "cleanser." In the wintertime, grow grass in pots indoors for your cat to nibble.

- Cats need water, especially when some of their food is dry, so always provide a supply of fresh water. Being of desert origin, cats have a different metabolism than dogs, so they can get by with less water.

- Never give a cat a commercial dog food. Cats need a different formula that's higher in protein and fat and lower in carbohydrates which can cause diabetes and other serious health problems when present in excess.

SAFETY HAZARDS

- If your cat goes outdoors, it should wear an identity tag.

- Be as vigilant with your kitten as with a child in safe-proofing the house. Be sure all window screens are secure and swing doors open and shut smoothly.

- If you have houseplants, make sure they're not poisonous to cats (like Dieffenbachia). Keep out of reach. Cats love to nibble plants.

- Close drawers and closets that contain needles, threads, pills, and other potentially harmful, swallowable objects.

- Be careful to lock away insecticides and other household chemical compounds, as well as automobile antifreeze.

- Keep electrical extension cords concealed or covered to help stop young animals from chewing through the wires and being electrocuted. Unplug when not in use.

REASONS FOR NEUTERING

- Female cats howl and cry, sometimes for hours, during heat and become difficult to handle in their desire to get out. The best solution is to spay your female.

- Spaying is a safe and relatively easy operation with few if any aftereffects.

- A spayed cat has less chance of having ovarian and mammary cancer or uterine problems later in life.

- Males, propelled by the sex urge, will roam the neighborhood and get into courtship fights. Also, mature males have a bad habit of spraying the house. The best solution is to neuter your male.

GOOD BREEDING

- Avoid inbreeding as much as possible if you are a cat breeder. Do not breed stress-susceptible, emotionally unstable animals, because these qualities can be passed on to the offspring. Ask for progeny records and screening for genetic defects and hereditary diseases.

• When buying a purebred, select a robust kitten. One that looks frail and appears excessively timid or nervous may well be a sickly and costly pet to keep. Good breeding contributes significantly to animal health and is one of the most important preventive health measures that is only too often overlooked.

• Mixed-breed "alley" cats are generally healthier than highly inbred animals. I call these super-cats "Natural" cats. Being purebred is to be unnatural because it entails exclusive intergenerational inbreeding that never occurs in nature to any significant degree. Similarly, extreme traits (like Pug dog and Persian cat pushed-in faces) are linked with health problems, behavioral and cognitive impairment, and lower viability and quality of life. (with, therefore, increased need for human care). Natural selection takes the opposite direction of such artificial (human) selection, toward increased fitness, viability, and health.

PROPER REARING

Kindness kills. A life without any stress can have adverse effects on an animal's health, because it would have little resistance if and when it is finally exposed to stress. A kitten raised in an overprotected environment by an overindulgent owner may, as an adult, have a sickly disposition and a poor stress tolerance.

My research shows that a little stress early in life helps young animals mature into stable, outgoing, and adaptable adults. Frequent handling and grooming, from early infancy on, and exposure to visual and auditory stimuli are beneficial. A very common stress reaction occurs when a young cat is taken to the vet's in the car for the first time. It may develop a high temperature simply from the stress of a first car trip! This obviously makes diagnosis more difficult.

Over-swaddled cats tend to become overdependent and over-attached to their owners. Then they overreact to separation when they are boarded or go to the groomer, for instance. The ensuing depression, anxiety, and refusal to eat food stress the body and increase the animal's susceptibility to disease.

If you can keep as close as possible to the following simple formula for feline health and well-being, you will enjoy a more mutually enhancing relationship, and face fewer disease and behavior problems:

Holistic Health =
  Right Breeding + Right Nutrition + Right Understanding
  and
  Relationship + Right Environment + Right Veterinary Attention.

These principles of holistic veterinary medicine are animals' rights, and their human companions' and caretakers' responsibility.

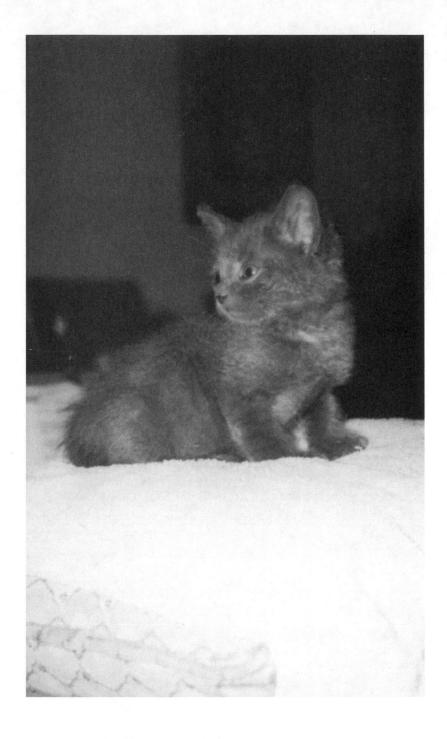

NATURAL HEALING

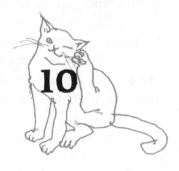

Throughout the recorded history of humankind, healers have used touch in various ways to alleviate sickness and suffering. Physical contact can range from the lightest touch, such as the laying on of hands, to deep and sometimes painful pressure to specific key areas of the body. In some of the more esoteric schools, the healer may go into an altered state of consciousness, a trance, or meditation. Or a healer may concentrate on the rhythm of her breathing, touching, or applying pressure as she breathes out, envisioning healing energy flowing through her hands. The inward breath, with hands still on the patient, draws in the sickness, which the healer bears and later shakes or washes off. This is a particular mind-set or imaginative/intuitive state of consciousness that is mentioned in a number of Eastern and Western schools of massage and healing, in which an attempt is made to coordinate the rhythm of one's own breathing with that of the patient.

It is regrettable that scientists, at least until recently, have refused to believe that nonphysical or nonmaterial phenomena that cannot be measured or quantified exist. Ideas and emotions exist, yet they are nonmaterial (unreal). While we do not have the scientific equipment to sense and record such phenomena, we do have minds and bodies to do so, and we can train our minds and bodies to become even more sensitively attuned and aware.

Indeed, a human being is an exquisitely sensitive instrument. Consider the vast range of sensory impressions that we take in when we look at someone or pet an animal. What limits this range are our beliefs, ideas, and expectations. If we believe that an animal doesn't really enjoy being touched and that its responses are mechanical and reflexlike, or if we massage each other or our pets in an unfeeling way, then there will be little or no benefit.

It is surprising to what degree the state of mind does influence the quality and effectiveness of the healing touch. This is a fact, verifiable through experience, yet it is an intangible and elusive challenge to scientific evaluation. It's rather like the placebo effect: The patient gets better if he or she believes in the doctor and the treatment the doctor prescribes. A doctor with the right positive attitude who believes in the treatment is more likely to facilitate the healing process via the placebo effect. The same holds true for massage therapy. This may all sound very esoteric or mystical, but it really isn't, once all of this is experienced and once one understands the healing power of the "physician within," which triggers the natural healing processes. This is the invisible art of medicine which modern, technological, drug-oriented, computerized, and depersonalized medicine has ignored at great cost to both patients and to the reputation of the medical profession. Fortunately, there has been a resurgence of interest in preventive, behavioral, and holistic medicine. And massage therapy is an integral part of this more integrative approach to health.

Massage therapy for cats is a "natural," since it can wholesomely exploit the close emotional bond between pet and owner. This does not rule out veterinarians and other qualified and experienced people from giving massage therapy to a cat. If the animal is used to being massaged from an early age, or has been well-handled and has been properly socialized to people, then there is no reason for the massage therapy not to be effective.

In addition, certain massage techniques have a direct effect upon the body and unconscious parasympathetic nervous system so that a patient who is unconscious, or one that might not initially believe in the benefits of massage therapy, is going to benefit anyway!

LIFE IS NATURAL ENERGY

The concept of energy fields and patterns within the body being disrupted by stress and sickness and balanced or restored through appropriate massage is common to several Eastern schools of massage. In Do-in massage therapy, for example, an oriental system based upon acupuncture principles, it is said that when a specific pressure point is sore or sensitive to the touch or spontaneously hurts, energy is in excess. Appropriate finger massage calms this accumulated or "jammed" energy.

It is generally believed by these Eastern schools that in addition to light, air, and food which nourish us, there also exist higher vibrations, electromagnetic energy called ki, or qi (which may be linked with positive and negative air ions), which the body captures through its many ki or pressure points. These points are skin deep, spirallic in structure, and dot the "meridians" or channels which transmit this electromagnetic energy throughout the body. This

energy is traditionally recognized as having two sources, the Yang
energy from the cosmos or sky and the Yin energy from the earth.
Note that the Indian points of the Chakras and Nadir correspond
to the Chinese acupuncture points, and their term for this energy is
also implicit in Prana, which comes from the Universal Mind and is
stored in the solar plexus. This is akin to such Christian concepts as
Divine Light, God, the Holy Spirit, and American Indian Great
White Spirit.

In good health, there is a free circulation of this life energy or ki,
coursing from organ to organ and from their corresponding meridians. Massage therapy helps eliminate blocks in the flow of this
energy, balancing and harmonizing the bioelectric field of mind and
body. In sickness, a blockage of ki causes an excess in certain parts
and deficiency in others which result in various disease symptoms.
Professor Namikoshi, a renowned Shiatsu teacher, states simply that
"The heart of Shiatsu is like pure maternal affection; the pressure of
the hands causes the springs of life to flow."

The healing touch (and the healing voice) benefit both the healer
and the patient, animal or human. As the physician within is acti-
vated in the animal or human, especially through touch, so in turn
are the physicians, pet owners, or masseurs, healing themselves in
the process!

I believe that the old injunction, "physician heal thyself," is
one of the extraordinary rewards of being a healer. And we can
all be healers, of animals and humans, because we all possess the
healing touch.

People of various cultures and at various times have referred to
this healing touch as vital energy, the life force, shakti (or shaktipat),
ki (or qi). It is possible to transmit and to feel this energy not only
through touch but also through eye contact. Animals are very sen-

sitive to this, because they use eye contact to establish dominance and to maintain social control.

Again referring to personal experience, I have, on more than one occasion, felt completely immersed in what I would describe as a bright, white light. During a laying-on-of-hands healing ritual, or while being blessed in a religious ceremony, people have seen and felt this energy, variously described as a "blinding flash," "ecstatic illumination," "the light of the Holy Spirit," or transfer of "chitti-shakti," the divine energy that gives life. What is especially intriguing to me is that people of different cultures and religions, past and present, have more or less the same sensory experience with this healing ray of light or energy that certain individuals can transmit! This is a challenge for science to objectively evaluate and quantify.

I do not consider this experience to be wholly beyond the realm of scientific inquiry or hypothetical probability, because modern physics has shown that all life and matter is energy. And one form of this energy is light, another touch. It is a fact, if not an oversimplification, that all living beings are complex bioelectric energy fields. Massage therapy, like the laying on of hands, is a form of energy exchange, whereby the patient may be literally re-energized and discordant energy patterns balanced—a process we call healing. Wellness is wholeness, rather than the absence of disease, as some Westernized physicians are trained to believe. And a potent and logical way to preserve this state of well-being is to maintain the right energy balances, as in the quality of food we eat and give our pets, the lifestyles we lead, and the quality of relationships we have. These especially can be stressful and not conducive to our overall well-being. Being emotionally deprived of the essential energy of another's affection is as bad as being deprived of some essential dietary nutrient. In fact, there are many physical, social, and emotional "nutrients," such as exercise and play and recreation, proteins and vitamins, affection, touch, and companionship, that are vital components of total health care for humans and nonhumans alike.

Young cats and other animals have been shown, like human infants, to waste away when not given affectionate contact. The tender loving touch is essential for the well-being and normal growth and development of all social animals because their bioelectric energy fields are dependent upon such input. As a seedling cannot thrive without the light of the sun, so, too, will we and our animal kin suffer without the energy of love.

RESTORING BALANCE

It is through touch especially, that this energy can be given and reciprocated. It is an essential part of our being. It helps us, through our relationships, stay whole and healthy. Having pets around to touch when we wish probably contributes more to our well-being than is generally realized. It probably contributes significantly to our pets' well-being, especially when there is only one pet and it has no companion animal to live with, groom, play with, etc. A regular massage for the pet can provide both pet and owner alike with that essential energy "nutrient" that is exchanged during touch and massage.

In sickness, when the ki is blocked (according to Eastern medical theory), energy imbalances are created. These lead to and reflect impaired functioning of various internal organs and body systems and can be corrected by manipulating certain ki points of access on the body surface. It is possibly through these same ki points that the healing light or energy of psychic healers operates. An indirect way of restoring balance in these energy systems is to give drugs, either homeopathically or allopathically, or work on the tissues and skeletal structures to bring about balance, through self-manipulation, as in yoga, or with a skilled manipulator, such as a chiropractor or Rolfer.

An additional human faculty of self-healing is through meditation or prayer. The former state may have its animal equivalent in that deeply passive and withdrawn state that sick cats will often go into, along with fasting.

In essence, Nature heals. Cats will eat grass, especially when they are "off color." Ancient peoples also observed what herbs other animals ate when they were sick, and then tried them themselves. Herbal medicine should soon become part of modern human and veterinary medicine as advances are made in integrating the various fields and specialties into the One Medicine (OM) of holistic health care and maintenance. There is and should only be one medicine, the basic principles of ease (health) and disease being the same for all creation, plant and animal, humans and cats. There may be subtle differences in the symptoms, necessitating slightly different approaches, but dehydration, lack of proper attention, malnutrition, and crowding stress are the same in many ways for a potted plant, a pet poodle, and a human being.

As we use the natural ways of different cultures to heal ourselves and our companion animals and discover new ways from nature, so we find the secret to health. It comes from living in harmony with ourselves, each other, and with nature as a whole: the quality of relationships influences our state of health as much as our temperament, perceptions, genetic constitution, and such. The same holds true for our animal companions.

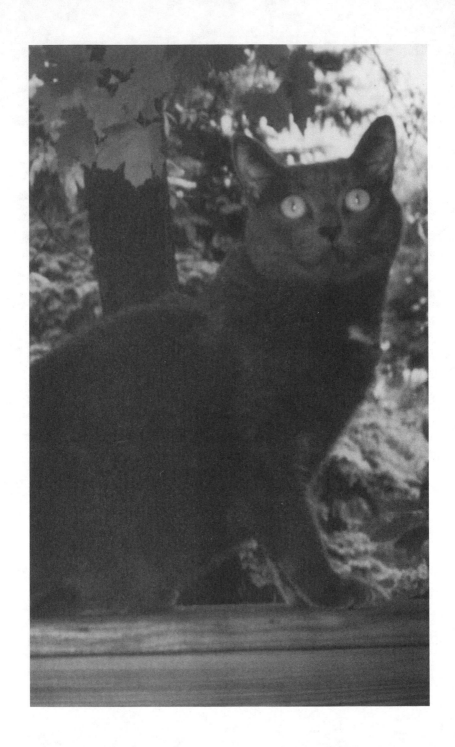

THE HEALING TOUCH
REVISITED

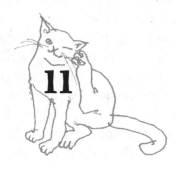

Before you contemplate massaging an animal, or giving any kind of treatment, you must first consider the fact that you are entering the animal's personal space. Even going to touch an animal, you must be mindful of your motives or intentions and sensitive to the condition, needs, and expectations of the other. Sometime it's best not to touch or to try giving a massage. Nothing of real benefit can be forced or imposed. What is most often best is usually gained through mutual accord.

With regard to caring for an animal, giving the Healing Touch, massage therapy, or other appropriate therapeutic procedure, the following tips are helpful: Provide a quiet, safe, soft-lighted space; a soft spot for the animal to lie on; reward intermittently with verbal praise or food treats. Burning incense relaxes many animals, as does a fine mist or heat haze of various natural essential plant oils like lavender and frankincense. Placing a little oil (diluted 30 drops per ounce of almond, hazel, or other light vegetable oil) on the animal's paws and ears and lightly on one's hands during the course of examination and treatment can help the animal learn to accept rewarding and beneficial contact and treatments through olfactory conditioning. It's best to let the animal choose which particular essential oil or combination thereof he or she prefers. Only use those they will sniff and not recoil from, and which they may lick or rub themselves against. These and other essential oils have beneficial influences, both physically and emotionally, and they are now being more widely used by holistic veterinarians in the United States, often in conjunction with other alternative therapies that are described in some of the books I have listed at the end of this essay.

The healing modalities of touch, and of smell, can be enhanced by the modality of sound. This has been virtually unexplored in Western medicine, the Muzak in doctors' and dentists' waiting rooms notwithstanding!

Various sounds and kinds of music help animals relax. Dairy farmers, for instance, use music to stimulate cows to let their milk down and relax prior to being milked. Animals, in turn, make various contentment sounds. Cats purr, dogs sigh and growl-groan during a massage.

Most animal sounds belong to the primal "paralanguage" of emotional conversation, which makes sense when our primal, aboriginal minds are connected!

Soft music where an animal is being examined or treated not only has a calming effect, it can also serve as a wall of sound to muffle sudden and disturbing noises outside and enhance the animal's sense of security. The tone of voice of the animal caretaker or therapist, mirrored in his or her body language, should convey a sense of calm, reassurance, and gentleness. In essence, it is more a question of how we speak to an animal than what we actually say, just as with giving the Healing Touch. It is more a question of how we give it than the particular technique we adhere to and may even, as some have done, trademark and market!

During my initial training in Swedish massage therapy under Naomi J. Leavitt at the San Mateo, California, Alpha Massage School, I was advised before giving a therapeutic massage to put aside my ego and surrender to the Higher Power so that I would not get in my own way as a sensitive care-giver. After I felt ill while massaging one student whose physical and emotional symptoms I took in and experienced myself, Naomi laughed and told me that was good and to be expected and that I should go and wash my hands. She also advised that, with time, I could learn to deal better with the "burden" and consequences of empathizing, provided I was able to let go and let be.

Before giving the Healing Touch or any beneficial treatment to another in need, a ritual is often done by many healers, some burning sage, praying, and chanting, others meditating or going into a more selfless state of awareness. Some fast between healings or engage in other forms of cleansing and balancing, from going into the woods with their dogs to practicing hatha yoga or other mind-body linking disciplines, like Chi-Kung and Tai-Chi. I wish all schoolchildren could be introduced to these psychophysical, mind-body integrating disciplines and be encouraged by enlightened elders.

When another being is receptive—openly trusting of what we hope to offer and may give selflessly for the other's good—we have the necessary foundation. Through the Healing Touch, which most all humans possess, we can enter a deeper, primal realm akin to communion, which we experience through loving kindness and express in compassionate action.

Sioux Medicine man Black Elk advised that, "Nothing will be

well unless we learn to live in harmony with the Power of the World as it lives and moves and does its work." This sacred power moves through all of life, and we humans have the ability to manipulate it to some extent, often with harmful consequences when our motivation is selfish, as with the suffering of animals who have been genetically engineered and cloned. Humans have the power of dominion, the power to dominate other beings, and to variously exploit them for selfish ends. But the higher power of loving kindness and compassionate action is what makes us humane. This power is the source and inspiration of the Healing Touch.

I have seen this power in action at India Project for Animals and Nature's (IPAN) Hillview Farm Animal Refuge in South India, where many animals at death's door have been brought back to life through tender loving care. This miraculous and sublime healing power of devoted service enables us to enter what I call the empathosphere—the realm in which we are emotionally connected and are aware of others' physical and emotional states. Devoted, compassionate service is the antithesis of animal veneration, in which there is no real empathy, and cows, elephants, and monkeys, for example, suffer because they are perceived only as sacred objects and are not treated as sentient subjects. Or else, as in the West, they are seen only as subjects of scientific investigation and economic exploitation. The Animal Refuge, founded and directed by Deanna Krantz, is IPAN's center of operations in The Nilgiris, Tamil Nadu, South India. (Visit the website at www.gcci.org and link to IPAN for more details). I have seen at IPAN's refuge how the power of love can heal seemingly incurable animal patients on whom the best of medicines and expert opinion have been tried and failed.

The Healing Touch can strengthen and revive an animal's spirit and will to live, and, on occasion, allow death to come with less fear and pain. The Healing Touch is transmitted through the medium of empathy, of a deep in-feeling for the other in need of relief from fear and pain, and from sickness in body, mind, and spirit.

The empathizer, or empath for short, can sense and feel the other's condition. The deeper the in-feeling, the greater the empath takes on and suffers the other's condition. Empathy involves intuitive understanding from which arises wisdom, bioethical sensitivity, and compassionate action.

Clinical detachment is no guarantee of protection and tends, as we see in our busy human and nonhuman hospitals today, to destroy the empathic connection between the caregivers and the ones in need.

In my experience, "immunization" (as distinct from desensitization) of the empath comes though compassionate action, of being able to do something immediate and most effective to help another living being in distress. To feel another's suffering and not be able to do anything about it is the cross of despair that every empath must bear.

The empath takes on, to varying degrees, the patient's symptoms and injuries, anguish, terror, and despair, ideally with growing resilience and understanding. This facilitates diagnostic interpretation of the other's symptoms and condition, and also helps in making a prognosis and deciding on the best course of treatment.

Some who give the Healing Touch may take on too much of others' suffering and begin to experience burnout. Often they feel alone because other people can't understand why they care and suffer so deeply. Father Matthew Fox speaks of empathic and compassionate people "receiving the stigmata of an Earth crucified" as they bear witness to the natural world being obliterated by the human species. The Serenity Prayer is most helpful in such circumstances, when one prays to the God of one's understanding or to one's Higher Power, to "Grant me the serenity to accept the things I cannot change, the courage to change the things I can, and the wisdom to know the difference."

This prayer is indispensable on countless occasions, from deciding when to euthanize an animal, to knowing and accepting your own limitations that impede the "Power of the World as it lives and moves and does its work," as Black Elk said.

The Healing Touch, in reviving and strengthening the animal's spirit and will to live, benefits the immune, circulatory, digestive, and other systems. Food for the spirit must be coupled with appropriate food and water for the body that is nourishing and pure.

Many domestic animals—shy cats, abused dogs, most adult wild animals— can tolerate little or no human contact or close presence. They teach us that we, as healers, handlers, and caretakers, must treat every animal as an individual and attune ourselves to their tolerances and intolerances. Being still and doing nothing may be the first step toward doing something for the animal when being still makes the animal less afraid, more curious, perhaps, and ultimately more accepting and approachable. Food reward and fresh water to drink can often facilitate this process, as can the Healing Touch once the animal accepts physical contact. Animals having wounds cleaned and bandages changed at IPAN's Animal Refuge rarely need to be forcibly restrained to stop them from struggling during these procedures. There is usually no need when one handler feeds the animal treats and another handler strokes and talks to the patient.

Most remarkable and informing was my witnessing on a daily basis how many of the resident animals who had been healed and given ample food and security would take care of newly arrived animals, acting especially attentive, gentle, and protective; and later, when appropriate, playful and socially accepting. The new animal being cared for often belonged to an entirely different species—I watched dogs caring for fawns and lambs; monkeys riding on cows and donkeys; billy goats sparring with young bulls; and young pups playing tag with a high-tailing calf.

The light of compassionate love is healing and life-affirming. These happy, caring animals at the Refuge helped restore the spirit and certainly speeded the recovery of the hundreds of sick and injured animals that IPAN's staff have taken in and healed. We came to accept and rely on these resident animals as our healing partners, and many of the dogs, cows, and older monkeys seemed to know it and acted accordingly.

PSYCHOPHYSICAL (MIND-BODY) CONSIDERATIONS

The importance of psychophysical activity (which is more than treadmill-type exercise) to the health and development of animals, and to their recovery from illness and injury, is not widely appreciated. Many of the health and behavioral problems of companion animals are due in part to a lack of varied psychophysical stimulation and activity, coupled with improper diet and too many unnecessary vaccinations and drug treatments, especially of steroids and pesticides.

Activities like playing together, running, swimming, chasing, chewing, and manipulating various toys and climbing (especially for cats); being trained with positive reinforcement; and being allowed to have some contact with the great outdoors (under safe and supervised conditions—no cat or dog should be allowed to roam free, away from homeowners) all contribute to an animal's health, to his or her overall well-being, and also to what I believe is the sense of self.

I feel deeply for the millions of animals that people keep as pets and who live a solitary life, often for hours in a crate or cage, never having any contact with their own species and little human contact during the workweek when no one is home.

The quality of life, sense of self, and general health of these isolated and deprived souls would be greatly enhanced by the presence of one or more compatible animals in the home. Only another kindred being can fill the emotional and social void of the solitary pet. Few human caretakers can do this very well.

One-cat, one-dog, one-parrot, or other one-pet households are likely to have higher veterinary bills and sicker animals than the two-dog or -cat home, or multiple animal species household. An animal living alone is deprived of the myriad psychophysical benefits of a same- or compatible-species playmate, companion, caregiver, or -receiver. The same is true for elephants and other circus and zoo caged animals, as well as the dogs, cats, monkeys, and other species incarcerated in commercial and biomedical research laboratories, and the billions of poultry, pigs, and other creatures confined and crowded in factory farms.

The Healing Touch can liberate all creatures great and small, because it enables us to connect our hearts and minds with their spirits for the good of all.

Those who develop their Healing Touch may become "sensitives," their intuitive senses opening to new dimensions of mind-body connectedness with the Earth and other living beings. Some become adept dowsers, kinesiologists, others more prescient, even prophetically clairvoyant. There are stories of great healers of the past whose mere presence could heal. Being present and bearing witness is the first step on the path toward health, wholeness, and harmony that I hope this book will help open and widen. Our animal companions are our mirrors in many ways. They can be our healers and teachers, too. Only ignorance, fear, and disbelief hold us back from life's embrace.

In order to find a veterinarian who shares these concerns and appreciates and applies the Healing Touch in the practice of empathic and holistic veterinary medicine, contact:

American Holistic Veterinary Association
2218 Old Emmorton Road
Bel Air, MD 21015
Visit www.ahvma.org

American Veterinary Chiropractic Association, Inc.
623 Main Street
Hillsdale, IL 61257
Visit www.avcadoctors.com

International Veterinary Acupuncture Society
PO Box 271395
Fort Collins, CO 80527-1395
Visit www.ivas.org

Veterinary Botanical Medicine Association
334 Knollwood Lane
Woodstock, GA 30188
Visit www.vbma.org

FURTHER READING

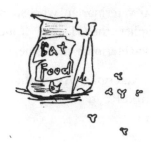

Anderson, Nina and Howard Peiper. *Are You Poisoning Your Pets?* East Canaan, CT: Safegoods, 1995.

Bell, Kristin Leigh. *Holistic Aromatherapy for Animals.* New York: Lantern Books, 2002.

Dossey, Larry. *Healing Beyond the Body: Medicine and the Infinite Reach of the Mind.* Boston: Shambhala, 2003.

Edalati, Rudy. *Barker's Grub: Easy, Wholesome Home-Cooking for Your Dog.* New York: Three Rivers Press, 2001.

Fox, Michael W. *The Boundless Circle: Caring for Creatures and Creation.* Wheaton, IL: Quest Books, 1996.

Fox, Michael W. *Bringing Life to Ethics: Global Bioethics for a Humane Society.* Albany, NY: State University of New York Press, 2001.

Fox, Michael W. *Eating With Conscience: The Bioethics of Food* Troutsdale, OR: NewSage Press, 1997.

Goldstein, Martin. *The Nature of Animal Healing.* New York: Knopf, 1999.

Kelleher, Donna. *The Last Chance Dog: And Other True Stories of Holistic Animal Healing.* New York: Scribner's, 2003.

McElroy, Susan Chernak. *Animals as Teachers and Healers, New Edition.* New York: Ballantine Books, 1998.

Martin, Ann N. *Food Pets Die For: Shocking Facts about Pet Food.* Troutdale, OR: NewSage Press, 2003.

Pitcairn, Richard J. and Susan Hubble Pitcairn. *Natural Health for Dogs and Cats.* Emmaus, PA: Rodale Press, 1995.

Schoen, Alan G. and Susan G. Wynn. *Complementary and Alternative Veterinary Medicine: Principles and Practice.* Indianapolis, IN: Mosby, 1998.

Snow, Amy, et al. *The Well-Connected Dog: A Guide to Canine Acupuncture.* Denver: Tall Grass Publishers, 1999.

Strombeck, Donald R. *Home-Prepared Dog and Cat Diets.* Ames, IA: Iowa State University Press, 1998.

Wynn, Susan G. *Emerging Therapies: Using Herbs and Nutraceuticals for Small Animals.* Lakewood, CO: American Animal Hospital Association, 1999.

Wynn, Susan G. and Steve Marsden. *Manual of Natural Veterinary Medicine.* St. Louis, MO: Mosby, 2002.

INDEX

(Page numbers in italics indicate pages with illustrations.)

U
uterine infections, 87

V
vaccinations, 111
veterinarians. *See also* health care
    for cats
  finding empathic/holistic
    practitioner, 137
  signs of need for, 110-11

W
whiskers, 53
wolf massage, ix-x
worming, 111-12

Y
Yin and Yang, 124

ACKNOWLEDGMENTS

My thanks to Esther Margolis for publishing my work, and to Theresa Burns, Keith Hollaman, and Shannon Berning for editing new material and for revising and recasting the earlier edition of *The Healing Touch* specifically for dogs and cats.

I wish to express my appreciation to the many veterinarians and other animal caregivers, and so many pet owners who have written to me, sharing their appreciation and experiences of applying the Healing Touch to their animal patients and companions. My lifelong aspiration as a veterinarian and animal behaviorist has always been to repair and restore the ancient bond of kinship between humans and other animals and the natural world, and I am grateful to Newmarket Press for contributing to this necessary unity by publishing my work.

ABOUT THE AUTHOR

Dr. Michael W. Fox graduated from the Royal Veterinary College, London, England, in 1962, earned a Ph.D. in medicine in 1967, and a D.Sc. in ethology/animal behavior from the University of London in 1976. Between 1967–1976 he was a professor at Washington University, St. Louis, Missouri, and subsequently worked in animal protection as an advocate of humane care, bioethics, holistic veterinary medicine, and conservation. His nationally syndicated newspaper column "Animal Doctor" with United Features reaches millions of readers, and he is the author of over 40 books on animal-related issues.

Dr. Michael W. Fox's Pet Care Books

The Healing Touch for Cats
This proven massage program for cats helps affirm the human-animal bond by providing instruction on why cats need massage, how to understand your cat's body language, how to give a diagnostic or therapeutic massage, and how to keep your cat healthy.

The Healing Touch for Dogs
Utilizing the same holistic philosophy of animal well-being, Dr. Fox teaches you basic dog psychology, how massage can help your dog, how to create the best massage routine, how to diagnose illnesses, and how to keep your dog in shape.

Love Is a Happy Cat
Cartoons by Harry Gans
Wonderfully and wittily illustrated, *Love Is a Happy Cat* "captures everything that is truly important about cat care and behavior in a handful of words" (*Cat Fancy*). If cats could write, here's what they would say about life and love.

The New Animal Doctor's Answer Book
Illustrated by B. J. Lewis
This fascinating sourcebook, drawn from Dr. Fox's nationally syndicated column, answers more than 1,000 questions about the health, psychology, and well-being of cats, dogs, fish, birds, rabbits, and other companion animals.

Ask for these titles at your local bookstore or use this coupon to order from Newmarket Press, 18 East 48th Street, New York, NY 10017.
Please send me:

_____Copies of *The Healing Touch for Cats* at $12.95
_____Copies of *The Healing Touch for Dogs* at $12.95
_____Copies of *Love Is a Happy Cat* at $6.95
_____Copies of *The New Animal Doctor's Answer Book* at $14.95

For postage and handling, add $4.00 for the first book ordered and $1.00 for each additional book. (New York State residents add applicable sales tax.) Allow 4-6 weeks for delivery. Prices and availability subject to change. (For credit card orders, call 800-669-3903.)
I enclose check or money order payable to NEWMARKET PRESS in the amount of $_____

NAME:_____

ADDRESS:_____

CITY/STATE/ZIP:_____

Special discounts are available for bulk orders. For information contact Newmarket Press, Special Sales Dept., 18 East 48th St., NY, NY 10017; phone 212-832-3575 or 800-669-3903; fax 212-832-3629; or e-mail mailbox@newmarketpress.com.

Website: www.newmarketpress.com